ON-CALL
in ENT
Surgery

Hannah R. Nieto
NIHR Academic Clinical Lecturer in ENT

Katherine McNamara
Higher Speciality Trainee in ENT

Samantha Goh
Higher Speciality Trainee in ENT

Nina Mistry
Post-CCT Otology Fellow

Shahram Anari
Consultant ENT Surgeon
University Hospitals Birmingham NHS Foundation Trust

Foreword by:
Professor Hisham Mehanna
Professor of Head and Neck Surgery, Institute for Head and Neck Studies
and Education, University of Birmingham, UK

Series editors:
Mr Karl F.B. Payne
Clinical Research Fellow, University of Birmingham
Specialty Trainee in Oral and Maxillofacial Surgery, West Midlands Deanery

Mr Arpan S. Tahim
Specialty Trainee in Oral and Maxillofacial Surgery, London Deanery

Mr Alexander M.C. Goodson
Head and Neck Fellow, Queen Elizabeth Hospital Birmingham

First published in 2020 by Libri Publishing

Copyright © Hannah Nieto, Katherine McNamara, Samantha Goh, Nina Mistry and Shahram Anari

The right of Hannah Nieto, Katherine McNamara, Samantha Goh, Nina Mistry and Shahram Anari to be identified as the authors of this work has been asserted in accordance with the Copyright, Designs and Patents Act, 1988.

ISBN 978-1-911450-72-6

A CIP catalogue record for this book is available from The British Library

Cover and Design by Carnegie Publishing

Printed in the UK by Halstan

Libri Publishing
Brunel House
Volunteer Way
Faringdon
Oxfordshire
SN7 7YR

Tel: +44 (0)845 873 3837

www.libripublishing.co.uk

CONTENTS

About the editorial team   viii

About the On-Call Series   ix

Dedication   x

Acknowledgements   xi

Abbreviations   xii

Foreword   xiv

Introduction   1

Disclaimer   2

Chapter 1: Essentials   **3**

    1.1 ENT in brief   3

    1.2 Referrals   4

    1.3 Anatomy   5

    1.3.1 Surface anatomy   5

    1.3.2 Nasal anatomy   6

    1.3.3 Sinus anatomy   7

    1.3.4 Temporal bone anatomy   7

    1.3.5 Facial nerve   7

    1.3.6 Ear   8

    1.3.7 Neck   9

    1.3.8 Thyroid / parathyroid and salivary gland   10

    1.3.9 Salivary glands   11

    1.3.10 Oral cavity   12

    1.4 ENT history taking   13

    1.4.1 Focussed history   13

    1.5 Clinical examinations   15

    1.5.1 Ear examination   15

    1.5.2 Tuning fork tests   16

    1.5.3 Free field hearing testing   17

    1.5.4 Neck examination   18

    1.5.5 Thyroid examination   20

    1.5.6 Nasal examination   22

1.5.7 Airway examination   23

1.6 Radiology   25

1.6.1 Lateral soft tissue neck x-ray   25

1.6.2 Computed tomography (CT) of the paranasal sinuses   27

1.6.3 Computed tomography (CT) of the temporal bone   28

1.7 Audiometry   30

1.7.1 Pure-tone audiogram   30

1.7.2 Tympanometry   31

1.8 ENT prescribing   33

1.8.1 Ear drops   33

1.8.2 Nasal drops   36

1.8.3 Saline nasal douching   38

1.8.4 Antibiotics   39

1.8.5 Nasal packing and topical agents   40

1.8.6 High-dose steroid prescribing   41

1.8.7 Nebulisers   43

Chapter 2: Emergency department   **45**

2.1 Acute airway compromise   45

2.2 Tonsillitis   48

2.3 Quinsy   50

2.4 Epiglottitis   52

2.5 Neck lump   54

2.6 Oesophageal foreign body   56

2.7 Ludwig's angina   58

2.8 Acute sialadenitis   60

2.9 Epistaxis   62

2.10 Periorbital cellulitis   64

2.11 Acute rhinosinusitis   66

2.12 Facial nerve palsy   68

2.13 Nasal foreign body   70

2.14 Ear foreign body   72

2.15 Tympanic membrane perforation   74

2.16 Acute otitis media   78

2.17 Acute mastoiditis   82

2.18 Otitis externa   85

2.19 Necrotising otitis externa   89

2.20 Acute vertigo   91

2.21 Sudden onset hearing loss   94

2.22 Perichondritis   96

2.23 Facial trauma and head injuries   97

2.24 Temporal bone fracture   99

2.25 Penetrating neck trauma   101

2.26 Blunt neck trauma   103

Chapter 3: Operating theatre   **105**

3.1 General principles   105

3.2 Specialist theatre equipment   107

3.2.1 Endoscopic surgery   107

3.2.2 Surgical microscope   107

3.2.3 Nerve monitors   108

3.2.4 Lasers   108

3.3 Consenting patients for theatre   110

3.3.1 Consenting patients   110

3.3.2 Complex consent situations   111

3.3.3 Arrest of post-tonsillectomy bleed   111

3.3.4 Manipulation under anaesthetic of fractured nose   112

3.3.5 Mastoidectomy (acute)   112

3.3.6 Tracheostomy   112

3.3.7 Drainage of septal haematoma   112

3.3.8 Nasal/ear foreign body removal   112

3.3.9 Rigid oesophagoscopy (+/- removal foreign body)   113

3.3.10 Drainage of periorbital abscess   113

3.3.11 Deep space neck abscess   113

3.3.12 SPA ligation   113

3.3.13 Grommet insertion   113

Chapter 4: Ward **115**

4.1 Post-op head and neck patients 115

4.1.1 Types of drain 115

4.1.2 Flap care 115

4.1.3 Parenteral feeding 116

4.1.4 Swallowing assessment 116

4.1.5 Post-operative thyroid patients 116

4.1.6 Tracheostomy care 117

4.1.7 Laryngectomy care 117

4.2 Post-op rhinology patients 119

4.2.1 Nasal packs 119

4.2.2 Nasal splints 119

4.2.3 Pituitary patients 119

4.3 Post-op otology patients 120

4.3.1 Head bandage and dressings 120

4.3.2 Packs 120

4.3.3 Aftercare 120

4.3.4 Basic post-op checks 121

4.4 Post-operative complications 122

4.4.1 Post-tonsillectomy or post-adenoidectomy bleed 122

4.4.2 Thyroid haematoma 123

4.4.3 Oesophageal perforation 124

4.4.4 Epistaxis after nasal surgery 124

4.4.5 Tracheostomy tube displacement 125

Chapter 5: Clinic **127**

5.1 Emergency clinic 127

5.2 Main ENT clinic 128

5.3 Subspecialist ENT clinics 129

5.3.1 Balance clinic 129

5.3.2 Head and neck clinic 129

5.3.3 Other specialist clinics 130

Chapter 6: Procedures   **133**

    6.1 Nasal cautery   133

    6.2 Nasal packing   134

    6.3 Quinsy drainage   136

    6.4 Pinna haematoma   137

    6.5 Septal haematoma drainage   138

    6.6 Flexible nasendoscopy   139

    6.7 Ear microsuction   141

    6.8 Foreign body removal   142

        6.8.1 Removal of a nasal foreign body   142

        6.8.2 Removal of an ear foreign body   143

        6.8.3 Removal of an oropharyngeal foreign body 143

    6.9 Changing a tracheostomy tube   145

    6.10 Laryngectomy patient speaking valves   148

    6.11 Nerve blocks of the nose and pinna   149

    6.12 Manipulation under anaesthetic (MUA) fractured nose   154

    6.13 Cricothyroidotomy   155

Author biographies   157

Bibliography   158

Index   159

ABOUT THE EDITORIAL TEAM

Mr Karl F.B. Payne

BMedSci(Hons) BMBS BDS MRCS

Clinical Research Fellow, University of Birmingham

Specialty Trainee in Oral and Maxillofacial Surgery, West Midlands Deanery

Mr Arpan S. Tahim

BSc (Hons) MBBS BDS MRCS MEd

Specialty Trainee in Oral and Maxillofacial Surgery, London Deanery

Mr Alexander M.C. Goodson

BSc(Hons) FRCS(OMFS) DOHNS

Head and Neck Fellow, Queen Elizabeth Hospital Birmingham

ABOUT THE ON-CALL SERIES

The "On-call" series is a unique learning resource consisting of concise, accessible and highly readable books. Authored and edited by a team with a strong focus on medical and surgical education, they have proven to be highly useful both for junior doctors seeking guidance early on in their clinical rotations and for those with more experience who are looking to consolidate and develop their knowledge. Written as "survival guides," each book covers common presentations in the emergency, ward and clinic settings, along with detailed step-by-step descriptions of typical surgical procedures. The attention to hands-on practical advice with easy to follow instructions mean they are the only handbooks that a junior trainee should not be without.

DEDICATION

This book is dedicated to Tilly, Tom, Nia, Rohan, Keith, Matilda, Tom, Peter, Rebecca, Lillian and Shervin. Thank you for supporting us through all the challenges and rewards a surgical career brings.

ACKNOWLEDGEMENTS

We would like to thank Mr Tom Saunders and Mr Duncan Bowyer for their help and the use of some of their images in this book. Thank you to Dr Akash Jangan for his assistance with the images. We would also like to thank Mr Chris Coulson and Mr Ajith George at endoscope-i for their images (Figure 21).

We would like to thank the Difficult Airway Society for their excellent guidelines and for allowing us to use their images in Figure 18 and Figure 35. These were reproduced from the Difficult Airway Society 2015 guidelines for management of unanticipated difficult intubation in adults (C. Frerk, V.S. Mitchell, A.F. McNarry, C. Mendonca, R. Bhagrath, A. Patel, E.P. O'Sullivan, N.M. Woodall and I. Ahmad, Difficult Airway Society intubation guidelines working group, *British Journal of Anaesthesia*, 115 (6): 827–848 (2015) doi:10.1093/bja/aev371) and are available with the guidelines on das. uk.com.

We acknowledge the use of an image (Figure 22) from NICE, subject to the following statements:

© NICE (2018) NG91 Otitis media (acute): antimicrobial prescribing. Available from

https://www.nice.org.uk/guidance/ng91/resources/visual-summary-pdf-4787282702

All rights reserved. Subject to Notice of rights.

NICE guidance is prepared for the National Health Service in England. All NICE guidance is subject to regular review and may be updated or withdrawn. NICE accepts no responsibility for the use of its content in this product/publication.

We acknowledge Elinor Carey for volunteering to model in this book and the fantastic images produced by Margaret Delaney-Quirke. Thanks go to the authors of *On-call in Oral and Maxillofacial Surgery*, especially Karl Payne, Arpan Tahim and Alexander Goodson, for allowing us to use their book images and for helping us shape the final version of this book.

ABBREVIATIONS

AC	air conduction
ANA	antinuclear antibodies
AOM	acute otitis media
AP	anteroposterior
ATLS	Advanced Trauma Life Support
BAETS	British Association of Endocrine and Thyroid Surgeons
BC	bone conduction
BIPP	bismuth iodoform paraffin paste
BNF	*British National Formulary*
BP	blood pressure
CHL	conductive hearing loss
CN	cranial nerve
CPA	cerebellopontine angle
CRP	C-reactive protein
CRS	chronic rhinosinusitis
CSF	cerebrospinal fluid
CT	computed tomography
DAS	Difficult Airway Society
dBHL	decibels hearing level
EAC	external auditory canal
EMG	electromyographic
ENOG	electroneuronography
ENT	ear, nose and throat (or "otorhinolaryngology")
EPOS	European Position Paper on Rhinosinusitis and Nasal Polyps
ESR	erythrocyte sedimentation rate
FB	foreign body
FBC	full blood count
FEES	fibre-optic endoscopic evaluation of swallowing
FESS	functional endoscopic sinus surgery
FNA	fine needle aspirate
HHT	hereditary haemorrhagic telangiectasia

Hib	*Haemophilus influenza* type b
Hz	hertz
IAM	internal auditory meatus
IPD	inter-pupillary distance
IV	intravenous
kg	kilogram(s)
MC&S	microscopy, culture and sensitivity
MDT	multidisciplinary team
mg	milligram(s)
MI	myocardial infarction
MRI	magnetic resonance imaging
MUA	manipulation under anaesthetic
NBM	nil by mouth
NCEPOD	National Confidential Enquiry into Patient Outcome and Death
NG	nasogastric
NICE	National Institute for Health and Care Excellence
NOE	necrotising otitis externa
OE	otitis externa
OGD	oesophago-gastro-duodenoscopy
PE	pulmonary embolism
PTA	pure-tone audiogram
SIGN	Scottish Intercollegiate Guidelines Network
SLT	speech and language therapist
SNHL	sensorineural hearing loss
SPA	sphenopalatine artery
T3	triiodothyronine
T4	thyroxine
TEP	transoesophageal puncture
TSH	thyroid stimulating hormone
U&Es	urea and electrolytes
USS	ultrasound scan

FOREWORD

Clinical practice has changed considerably for trainees over the last decade. Much of that has been positive, with increasing emphasis on evidence-based treatment, patient safety and the quality of care. Some changes, however, have not been positive, such as the loss of the "firm" structure, and the inevitable introduction of partial shift rotas, which often have led to an interruption in the continuity of training.

Junior clinicians and trainees are most exposed during their on-calls. They can be the first port of call for a wide variety of conditions, some of which are urgent. They may not need to manage these cases themselves, but they need to be able to recognise those conditions and when to call for assistance.

Therefore, never has there been a more important time for trainees and junior doctors, practising and treating patients in otorhinolaryngology departments, to be up to date with the basics *and* the details of the management of emergency patients presenting to the on-call team.

This excellent book, from a team of dedicated trainees, elucidates all that is needed. Covering all topics, from anatomy all the way to the details of management, it is comprehensive, clear and concise.

I wish that I could have had something like this when I was starting out myself as an ENT trainee. I thoroughly recommend it!

Prof Hisham Mehanna

PhD, BMedSc (hons), MB ChB (hons), FRCS, FRCS (ORL-HNS)
Professor of Head and Neck Surgery

Deputy Pro-Vice Chancellor (Interdisciplinary research)

Director, The Institute for Global Innovation (I.G.I.) & the Institute for Advanced Studies (I.A.S), University of Birmingham

Director, Institute of Head and Neck Studies and Education (InHANSE)

INTRODUCTION

ENT surgery is a speciality that manages acute and chronic presentations of ear, nose, throat, and head and neck conditions. It is difficult to cover all aspects of ENT in undergraduate training due to the extent of the subspecialties it encompasses. This can understandably leave junior doctors feeling apprehensive when commencing an ENT rotation or cross cover.

This book acts as both a survival guide for newcomers to the speciality and a reference for more experienced junior trainees. It covers everything from emergency presentations to minor surgical procedures and captures the fascinating nature of the speciality. We hope you enjoy the book as much as we have enjoyed writing it!

H.N., K.M., S.G., N.M., S.A.

DISCLAIMER

This book is not a textbook but is designed to be a survival guide. All content has been written by the authors and is obtained from reliable sources and personal experience. The authors and publishers do not accept responsibility or legal liability for injury or damage to any person as a result of action or refraining from action due to the clinical material in this book. At the time of printing, the drug doses contained within this book were correct, but it is the reader's responsibility to check up-to-date manufacture and drug dose safety guidelines.

CHAPTER 1: ESSENTIALS

1.1 ENT IN BRIEF

Otorhinolaryngology (ENT) covers several subspecialities, including otology, rhinology, facial plastics, head and neck, and paediatric ENT. ENT specialists manage a variety of conditions that require a multidisciplinary approach from allied healthcare providers such as speech and language therapists, audiologists, and vestibular physiotherapists. The MDT approach also extends to the involvement of other surgical and non-surgical specialities. Maxillofacial, vascular and plastic surgeons and oncologists regularly assist head and neck surgeons with management of their patients (e.g. reconstruction with flaps and microvascular anastomosis). Rhinologists, specifically anterior skull base surgeons, often work closely with neurosurgeons to perform pituitary procedures that are then managed post-operatively alongside endocrine physicians.

Management of ENT patients can sometimes be daunting for new junior doctors as some conditions and procedures are not commonly encountered outside of ENT. ENT is a speciality that often allows junior doctors to manage patients independently in the A&E and outpatient setting. This, together with the practical nature of the speciality, makes it very rewarding and a great place to learn new skills (see Chapter 6: Procedures). This current chapter will introduce some of the key principles involved in managing ENT patients.

1.2 REFERRALS

When receiving a referral, it is important to determine the clinical suspicion and a provisional management plan from the referrer. The majority of ENT referrals are non-urgent and suitable for an emergency clinic appointment. It is therefore important to obtain the patient details (including name, date of birth, NHS number and a telephone number) as well as the name and contact details (telephone number) of the referring clinician. This enables discussion of the case with a senior if there is any doubt as to how to triage the patient. For any referrals involving the throat or neck, always clarify whether or not the patient has any airway compromise and whether or not they are haemodynamically stable. Table 1 below categorises some key ENT conditions and how to triage them.

Attend and review immediately	Review in A&E	Appropriate for ENT emergency clinic (see within a week)	Appropriate for ENT main consultant clinic
Stridor (advise caller to also call anaesthetist on-call)	Tonsillitis/quinsy	Facial nerve palsy (lower motor neurone, non-traumatic)	Concerns about underlying malignancy (two-week-wait referral)
Thyroid haematoma	Periorbital cellulitis	Fractured nose	Vertigo (see patient outside acute episode; if concerned about acute stroke, ask referrer to refer to the medical team urgently)
Ongoing epistaxis (advise caller to apply first aid)	Mastoiditis	Ear foreign bodies (battery – see urgently)	
Post-tonsillectomy or post-adenoidectomy bleed	Enlarging neck lump	Otitis externa	
	Oesophageal or nasal foreign bodies (battery – see immediately)	Acute hearing loss (see within 24 hours of onset)	Recurrent acute otitis media
Epiglottitis or supraglottitis	Facial trauma	Minor recurrent epistaxis (not actively bleeding)	Longstanding ENT conditions
Ludwig's angina	Temporal bone fracture	Sinusitis	
Neck trauma			

Table 1: Triaging referrals
There may be phone advice to give to the referring clinician, which is detailed in the emergency department chapter (Chapter 2).

ESSENTIALS

1.3 ANATOMY

1.3.1 SURFACE ANATOMY

The ability to describe the normal surface anatomy of the ear and nose is important in ENT (Figure 1). This will allow you to convey the location of the injury over the telephone to your senior effectively. Secondly, any patient who has facial injuries as a consequence of assault requires accurate documentation of those injuries as their notes will be used in any legal case that ensues.

ESSENTIALS

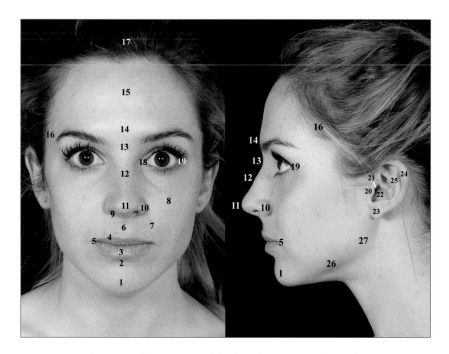

Figure 1: Facial view and key anatomical landmarks: 1 – mental protuberance; 2 – vermillion border; 3 – lower lip vermillion; 4 – upper lip vermillion; 5 – lateral commissure of lip; 6 – philtrum; 7 – nasolabial fold; 8 – cheek; 9 – anterior nares; 10 – alar; 11 – nasal tip; 12 – rhinion; 13 – nasion; 14 – glabella; 15 – forehead; 16 – temporal region; 17 – hairline; 18 – medial canthus; 19 – lateral canthus; 20 – tragus; 21 – incisura terminalis; 22 – concha; 23 – lobule; 24 – helical rim; 25 – antihelix; 26 – inferior border of the mandible; 27 – angle of mandible

1.3.2 NASAL ANATOMY

Flexible nasendoscopy allows a detailed assessment of the internal nose and postnasal space (Figure 2). Vascular anatomy of the internal nose is important in understanding the management of epistaxis, with five vessels supplying Kiesselbach's plexus in Little's area on the septum (Figure 3). This area is the source of most anterior nosebleeds.

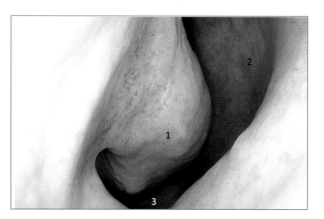

Figure 2: Right anterior nasal passage – view from inserting Thudichum nasal forceps or at start of nasendoscopy: 1 – inferior turbinate; 2 – nasal septum (Little's area); 3 – floor of nasal cavity

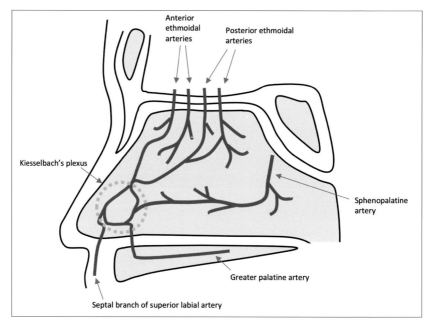

Figure 3: Key vessels supplying the nasal septum. The area of vessel confluence anteriorly is called Kiesselbach's plexus and is found anatomically in Little's area on the nasal septum.

1.3.3 SINUS ANATOMY

The paranasal sinuses are assessed using CT with the coronal views being most important. The sinuses should be well aerated (black on CT scan), with mucosal thickening, polyps and masses demonstrated as opacification (grey on CT scan). These are explored further in section 1.6.2.

1.3.4 TEMPORAL BONE ANATOMY

Understanding temporal bone anatomy is key to understanding middle ear operations, but this is a complex topic. Figure 4 below demonstrates key landmarks used in ear surgery (both emergency and elective).

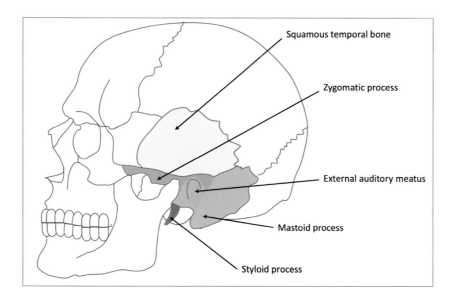

Figure 4: Constituent parts of temporal bone

1.3.5 FACIAL NERVE

The facial nerve travels through the middle ear and parotid gland, before dividing into the five motor branches demonstrated below in Figure 5. The anatomical course of the facial nerve is important in all presentations of facial nerve palsies: central (brain) and peripheral (middle ear, parotid origin) causes should be considered.

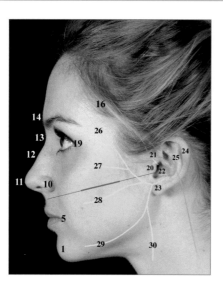

Figure 5: Branches of facial nerve: 26 – temporal branch; 27 – zygomatic branch; 28 – buccal branch; 29 – marginal mandibular branch; 30 – cervical branch; red line – location of parotid duct

1.3.6 EAR

The external ear is a cartilaginous structure; it is made up of various convexities and concavities (Figure 5). The lobule is the only part of the external ear where cartilage is absent. The external auditory canal (EAC) extends from the conchal bowl and ends at the tympanic membrane. The middle ear incorporates the ossicles, which conduct sound from the tympanic membrane to the cochlear, via the oval window (Figure 6). The lateral third of the EAC is cartilaginous and the medial two-thirds of the EAC is bony. At the medial end of the EAC sits the tympanic membrane (ear drum).

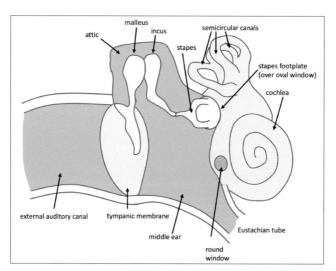

Figure 6: Middle ear anatomy – location of the ossicles beyond the tympanic membrane and connection to the inner ear (cochlea)

The tympanic membrane is made up of three layers: an external layer of skin, a middle layer of collagen and an internal mucosal layer. It is divided into two parts: a pars tensa inferiorly and a pars flaccida superiorly, the latter of which overlies the attic region (Figure 7). Structures of the middle ear such as the handle of the malleus can be visualised through the tympanic membrane on otoscopy. Sometimes additional structures such as the incudostapedial joint can be seen through a thin drum.

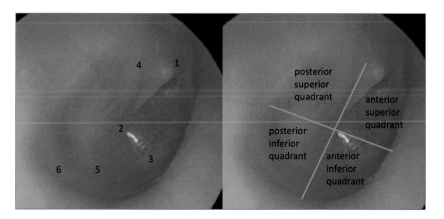

Figure 7: Normal right tympanic membrane: 1 – lateral process of the malleus; 2 – umbo; 3 – light reflex; 4 – pars flaccida; 5 – pars tensa; 6 – annulus

1.3.7 NECK

The neck is a complex structure made up of muscles, lymph nodes, vessels, lymphatic drainage, salivary glands, endocrine glands and the upper aerodigestive tract. Figure 8 shows the important surface anatomy of the neck, and the lymph node levels are described in Table 2. Both the triangles of the neck and the lymph node levels (primarily used for staging head and neck cancers) can be used to describe lesions or masses in the neck in the acute setting.

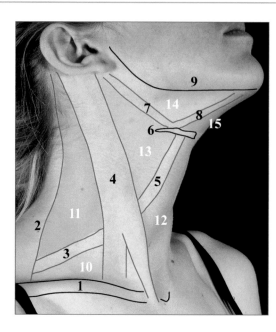

Figure 8: Important neck structures that define the triangles in the neck: 1 – clavicle (medially suprasternal notch); 2 – anterior border of trapezius; 3 – inferior belly of omohyoid; 4 – sternocleidomastoid muscle; 5 – superior belly of omohyoid; 6 – hyoid bone; 7 – posterior belly digastric muscle; 8 – anterior belly digastric muscle; 9 – inferior border mandible; 10 – supraclavicular triangle; 11 – occipital triangle; 12 – muscular triangle; 13 – carotid triangle; 14 – submandibular triangle; 15 – submental triangle

LEVEL I	Submental/submandibular triangle
LEVEL II	Skull base to inferior hyoid
LEVEL III	Inferior hyoid to inferior cricoid
LEVEL IV	Inferior cricoid to suprasternal notch
LEVEL V	Posterior triangle, posterior sternocleidomastoid to anterior trapezius
LEVEL VI	Central compartment, hyoid to suprasternal notch
LEVEL VII	Paratracheal nodes

Table 2: Lymph node levels in the neck

1.3.8 THYROID / PARATHYROID AND SALIVARY GLAND

1.3.8.1 THYROID GLAND

The thyroid is a butterfly shaped endocrine organ located in the midline of the neck, anteroinferior to the larynx. It synthesises triiodothyronine (T3) and thyroxine (T4) in response to thyroid stimulating hormone (TSH) from the pituitary gland. T3 and, to a lesser extent, T4 function peripherally on many organ sites, predominantly driving human metabolism. The embryological origin of the thyroid gland is the foramen caecum, which is found at the boundary of the anterior two-thirds and posterior third of the tongue. It descends into the neck during foetal development to rest in its final position over the third and fourth tracheal rings. The recurrent laryngeal nerves are found either side of the thyroid gland in the tracheal-oesophageal grooves; the right nerve runs at more of an oblique angle compared to the left. They enter the larynx at the level of the cricothyroid joints.

1.3.8.2 PARATHYROID GLANDS

The parathyroid glands are endocrine glands that are important in calcium homeostasis. There are usually four parathyroid glands, although this can range from two to six in some cases. The superior parathyroid glands originate from the fourth branchial arch and usually sit posteriorly to the recurrent laryngeal nerve and inferior thyroid artery. The inferior parathyroid glands originate from the third branchial arch descending into the neck with the thymus gland; for this reason their position is less consistent.

1.3.9 SALIVARY GLANDS

The main salivary glands within the head and neck consist of three pairs: the parotid, submandibular and sublingual glands (Figure 9).

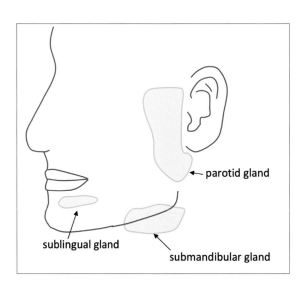

Figure 9: Diagram demonstrating location of salivary glands (all bilateral pairs)

ESSENTIALS

1.3.9.1 PAROTID GLANDS

The parotid glands are located laterally on the face, anterior and inferior to the pinna. They are divided into superficial and deep lobes by the facial nerve and retromandibular vein. The gland secretes serous watery saliva into the Stenson ducts, which open into the oral cavity adjacent to the second upper molars.

1.3.9.2 SUBMANDIBULAR GLANDS

These paired glands are located under the mandible in the submandibular triangle. The submandibular glands secrete a mixed mucus and serous saliva into Wharton's ducts, which enter the floor of the mouth at the lingual frenulum. The lingual, hypoglossal and marginal mandibular nerves lie in close proximity to the submandibular glands and are important to consider when performing submandibular gland excision.

1.3.9.3 SUBLINGUAL GLANDS

These glands are located in the floor of the mouth under the tongue and are the smallest of the named salivary glands. The secretions, which are mostly mucus, are secreted into multiple sublingual ducts which open into the sublingual folds.

1.3.10 ORAL CAVITY

- The oral cavity is the start of the digestive tract; it consists of the area between the oral fissure and the oropharynx.
- The oral cavity consists of the anterior two-thirds of the tongue, the upper and lower alveolus, 32 teeth in adults, the buccal mucosa, the hard palate and the floor of mouth.
- Key structures are labelled in Figure 10.

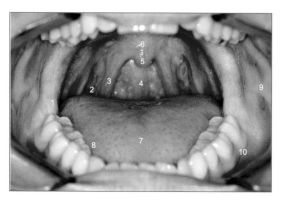

Figure 10: Oral cavity and oropharynx: 1 – retromolar trigone; 2 – palantine tonsil; 3 – palatopharyngeus; 4 – posterior pharyngeal wall; 5 – uvula; 6 – soft palate; 7 – tongue; 8 – lateral border of tongue; 9 – buccal mucosa; 10 – gingiva

1.4 ENT HISTORY TAKING

1.4.1 FOCUSSED HISTORY

1.4.1.1 PRESENTING COMPLAINT

Start with the presenting complaint and consider the points in Table 3.

EAR	Hearing loss: sudden/progressive/unilateral/bilateral
	Tinnitus: unilateral/bilateral/pulsatile/non-pulsatile
	Vertigo: rotatory/episodic/length
	Otalgia: sharp/dull/superficial/deep/constant/intermittent
	Otorrhoea: purulent/clear
NOSE	Nasal obstruction: unilateral/bilateral
	Epistaxis: which side/anterior or posterior
	Anosmia: conductive/sensorineural
	Rhinorrhoea: purulent/clear
	Postnasal drip
	Facial pain
THROAT	Odynophagia
	Dysphagia: solids/liquids
	Dysphonia: constant/intermittent
	Weight loss: time period
	Referred otalgia
	Chronic cough/haemoptysis
	Gastro-oesophageal reflux
	Neck lumps

Table 3: ENT history of presenting complaint

ESSENTIALS

1.4.1.2 PAST MEDICAL HISTORY

Does the patient suffer with any other medical conditions?

- Relevant to ENT: previous head and neck cancers, including dates and treatment, previous ENT/head-and-neck operations
- Risks for GA including cardiac disease, previous DVT/PE, respiratory disease

1.4.1.3 MEDICATION HISTORY

Does the patient take any medications? Do they have any allergies (drug allergy, aeroallergy, food allergy e.g. nut allergy)?

1.4.1.4 SOCIAL HISTORY

- Smoking history (pack years)
- Alcohol intake (units)
- Employment
- Family/support network (particularly in suspected head and neck cancers)
- Religious beliefs (e.g. objection to blood transfusion if Jehovah's witness)

1.5 CLINICAL EXAMINATIONS

1.5.1 EAR EXAMINATION

Begin by introducing yourself to the patient and obtaining verbal consent. Start by examining the better-hearing ear.

Inspection:

- Stand side-on to the patient
- Examine the pinna – from front and behind
- Look for skin inflammation, discharge, scars (endaural and postauricular) and skin lesions (pre-auricular sinus, skin tumours).

Palpation:

- Palpate the pinna and feel in front and behind the pinna for any pre- and postauricular lymph nodes, swelling over the mastoid.

Examine the external ear canal:

- Use an otoscope or a speculum and headlight
- Ask the patient if they have any pain
- Gently pull ear back and out (and upwards in adults)
- Look for inflammation, oedema, wax, discharge
- Visualise the tympanic membrane (Figure 7):
  - o Examine in quadrants, starting at 12 o'clock in the attic region
  - o Note the status of the tympanic membrane:
    - o Normal or dull
    - o Air bubbles – middle ear effusion (glue ear)
    - o Thin or tympanosclerotic (scarred)
    - o Perforation – which quadrant and what size (use estimated percentage of drum)
    - o Retraction pockets
    - o Visible ossicles
    - o Presence of grommets
    - o Debris/keratin

ESSENTIALS

- If a mastoid cavity is present, assess the following:
  - o Shape
  - o Size
  - o Dry (stable) or wet
  - o Remnant of tympanic membrane
  - o Presence and size of meatoplasty (widening of ear canal).

Pneumatic otoscopy/Valsalva on otoscopy can be used to assess middle ear function.

Fistula test – if the patient gives a history of dizziness/vertigo, this test can be performed by applying intermittent digital pressure to the tragus and observing the eyes for nystagmus. It is used to detect an abnormal connection (perilymph fistula) between the air-filled middle ear and the fluid-filled inner ear.

Completing the ear examination:

- Check facial nerve function
- Examine the postnasal space with an endoscope, especially if the patient has a unilateral middle ear effusion – this is in order to rule out the presence of malignancy
- Examine the remaining cranial nerves
- Perform tuning fork tests and free field hearing (detailed in sections below)
- Ask for a formal audiogram.

1.5.2 TUNING FORK TESTS

Rinne's and Weber's tests should be performed (Figure 11).

Rinne's test

- Compares air conduction (AC) vs. bone conduction (BC).

- Strike tuning fork (use a 512Hz tuning fork)

- Place alternately on mastoid process and external auditory meatus (EAM)

- Ask patient which is loudest

Interpretation of results:

Normal:

Positive Rinne – louder at EAM, AC > BC

Abnormal

True negative Rinne – louder on mastoid (BC > AC) = CHL

Positive Rinne – bilateral SNHL (AC > BC)

False-negative – severe unilateral SNHL, BC > AC, sound transmitted through skull to contralateral cochlear of better hearing ear

The Rinne test will detect CHL in 50% of patients with an air-bone gap of 20dB and 90% of patients with air-bone gap of 40dB

Weber's Test

- Uses bone conduction (BC) only

- Tests lateralization of sound

- Place the tuning fork in the midline of head, usually performed on the forehead

- Normal hearing or equal hearing loss – sound central

- Unilateral conductive loss – sound to poorer ear

- Unilateral SNHL – sound to better ear

Figure 11: Weber's and Rinne's tuning fork tests.

1.5.3 FREE FIELD HEARING TESTING

This is a "bedside" test and serves as a good adjunct to the audiogram, or as an alternative if audiogram not available. It can be done to give some idea of hearing loss. It is performed as follows:

- Turn patient's head to side (so the patient cannot see the examiner's mouth)

- Apply tragal rub masking to non-test ear

- Whisper at arm's length (60 cm), then increase loudness of voice in increments

- Patient to repeat the spoken numbers or words (these should be bisyllabic)
- If there is no response, the examiner can move closer (15 cm) from the ear and repeat the test
- To pass, the patient must repeat at least 50 % of the numbers or words correctly.

If the patient can hear a whisper at arm's length this indicates that hearing is likely to be normal. Hearing a normal voice at arm's length (but not the whisper) suggests a mild/moderate hearing loss. If the patient can only hear a loud voice at arm's length, this indicates a moderate/severe loss, whereas only being able to hear a loud voice close up suggests a profound loss. An indication of dB hearing loss at varying voice levels is shown in Table 4.

Voice Level	Distance	dB
Whisper	60 cm	12
	15 cm	34
Conversation	60 cm	48
	15 cm	56
Loud	60 cm	76

Table 4: Free field hearing testing dB hearing loss. Hearing sound below 20 dB is considered normal.

1.5.4 NECK EXAMINATION

In this section we cover examinations of the oral cavity, pharynx, larynx and neck. Thyroid examination and assessment of thyroid status are also included.

Examination of the oral cavity, pharynx and larynx (including nasendoscopy):

- Introduce yourself and obtain verbal consent for the examination.
- If the patient wears dentures, ask the patient to remove them.
- Use a headlight and have a tongue depressor available.
- Ask the patient to open their mouth widely – any restriction could be due to trismus.
- Inspect the tongue (dorsal/ventral and lateral aspects), dentition, gums (including the retromolar trigones) and the general state of the oral mucosa (white/red patches, ulcers).
- Inspect the hard and soft palates, palatine tonsils, uvula and posterior pharyngeal wall. Assess palatal elevation by asking the patient to say "ah".

- Use a gloved finger to palpate any areas that may have associated pathology and perform bi-manual palpation of the floor of the mouth with a gloved finger and a hand on the neck in the submandibular area.
- Examination of the rest of the pharynx (nasopharynx and hypopharynx) and larynx can be done using a flexible nasendoscope (see section 6.6).

Examination of the neck

Ensure the patient is sat upright in a chair and that you can gain access to the neck from behind the patient. Adequate exposure of the neck is important prior to commencing the examination.

Inspection:

- Look from the front and assess the neck for any scars, asymmetry or masses.
- Ask the patient to swallow and examine for any midline/thyroid masses rising on swallowing.
- If a midline mass is noted, ask the patient to open their mouth and then protrude the tongue. If the mass rises, it is more likely to represent a thyroglossal cyst.

Palpation:

- Ask the patient if they have any pain prior to commencing palpation of the neck.
- Standing behind the patient, assess all levels of the neck in a systematic manner (see Figure 8).
- Note the presence of any masses or lymphadenopathy.
- If a neck lump is palpated, assess the following: site, size, consistency, shape, pulsation, state of the overlying skin and fixity. The likely diagnosis can often be predicted based on the anatomical location of the lump (see Table 5).

Auscultation/percussion

- A stethoscope can be used to assess for the presence of bruits.
- Percussion may reveal evidence of retrosternal dullness secondary to a large thyroid mass.

ESSENTIALS

Sites	Potential diagnoses
Sublingual (level I)	Sublingual gland swelling or mass, lymph nodes
Submandibular (level II)	Submandibular gland swelling or mass, lymph nodes, dental abscess
Carotid region (level III)	Branchial cleft cyst, carotid body tumour, glomus tumour, lymph nodes
Supraclavicular (level IV)	Supraclavicular lymph node (left side – can be from GI pathology)
Posterior triangle (level V)	Lymph node, lipoma
Midline (Level VI)	Thyroid nodule or goitre, thyroglossal cyst, dermoid cyst
Pre-auricular	Pre-auricular sinus, parotid gland swelling or mass
All sites	Lymph nodes/lymph node mass (infective, inflammatory, malignancy), lipoma, haematoma, skin cancers

Table 5: Neck masses – diagnoses by site. See Figure 8 for demonstration of anatomical subsites.

1.5.5 THYROID EXAMINATION

Thyroid examination warrants further discussion as, although it includes a full neck examination, an assessment of thyroid status should also be performed.

- Examine the patient's face and hands and look for any features of hypo-/hyperthyroidism (Table 6).
- Whilst at the hands, feel for the patient's pulse and check for tachycardia (hyperthyroidism).
- Assess the eyes – look for features of Graves' disease (hyperthyroidism) – exophthalmos, lid retraction, proptosis, lid lag, chemosis and ophthalmoplegia.
- Examine the anterior neck and assess for obvious masses/scars and ask the patient to swallow – the thyroid gland moves with swallowing but not with protrusion of the tongue.
- Ask the patient whether they have any pain and begin palpation of the neck standing behind the patient.
- Palpate in the midline and ask the patient to swallow to help identify the thyroid. Most normal thyroids are not palpable.

- Assess each lobe as well as the midline isthmus in turn and make note of any lumps and describe as stated above.
- Complete palpation by assessing all remaining levels of the neck to check for lymphadenopathy.
- Auscultation/percussion: a stethoscope can be used to assess for the presence of a thyroid bruit.
- Percussion may reveal evidence of retrosternal dullness secondary to a large thyroid mass.

Hyperthyroidism	Hypothyroidism
Symptoms:	Symptoms:
Heat intolerance	Dry skin
Nervousness and irritability	Thinning hair
Muscle weakness	Constipation
Increased frequency of stools	Cold intolerance
Increased appetite	Hoarseness
Increased sweating	Reduced sweating
Restlessness	Tiredness
Fatigue	Paraesthesia
Blurred or double vision	Periorbital puffiness
Palpitations	Menstrual irregularities
Sleep disturbance	
Menstrual irregularities	
Signs:	Signs:
Tremor	Reduced mental function
Distracted attention span	Weight gain
Weight loss	Slowing of ankle jerk
Tachycardia	Slow movement
Goitre	Goitre
Hyperreflexia	Bradycardia
Proptosis	

Table 6: Signs and symptoms of hyper- and hypothyroidism

ESSENTIALS

ESSENTIALS

1.5.6 NASAL EXAMINATION

- Introduce yourself to the patient and obtain consent for the examination.
- Use a headlight.
- Inspect the nose externally from the front and lateral aspects: identify any scars, lesions or masses and note the skin quality. Look for asymmetry of the nasal bones/cartilaginous dorsum.
- Ask the patient to tilt their head back to assess the columella (scars, asymmetry, dislocation) and look for any obvious pathology in the nasal vestibule.
- Ask about pain prior to palpation. Feel the nasal bones and nasal cartilages for any asymmetry/deformity.
- Anterior rhinoscopy – use nasal Thudichums to assess the anterior nose – inspect the nasal vestibule (masses, lesions, inflammation), anterior septum (prominent vessels, deviation, haematoma, abscess), nasal mucosa, inferior turbinates (hypertrophy, inflammation), nasal polyps and masses.
- Use a metal tongue depressor under the nose to assess airway patency.
- Perform flexible nasendoscopy to examine the rest of the nasal cavity including the postnasal space (see below).
- Examine the neck for lymphadenopathy.

1.5.6.1 RIGID AND FLEXIBLE NASENDOSCOPY TO ASSESS THE NOSE

Rigid endoscopes are often used in ENT for examination and diagnostic purposes. A 0-degree Hopkins rod can be used to examine the nose as an alternative or in addition to the flexible nasendoscope. It can be used in conjunction with suction to allow thorough assessment of the nose as follows.

- Explain the nature of the procedure to the patient.
- Apply topical local anaesthetic spray to both sides of the nose.
- Lubricate the distal portion of the scope and introduce through the nose (do not lubricate the distal tip as this may obscure the view).
- Use a "three-pass" technique to assess the nose in a systematic manner:
    - o Pass the scope along the floor of the nose and through to the nasopharynx (Figure 2);
    - o Pass the scope under the middle turbinate to assess the middle meatus;
    - o Pass the scope medially to assess the surface of the middle turbinate and observe the roof of the nasal cavity.

- Assess the following: health of the nasal mucosa, turbinates, presence of mucopus, nasal polyps, masses, septal perforation and postnasal space (masses, adenoids, Eustachian tube openings).

All of the above is commonly performed using a flexible nasendoscope in clinic (Figure 12).

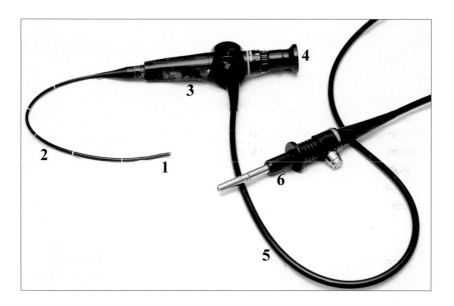

ESSENTIALS

Figure 12: Flexible nasendoscope: 1 – nasendoscope tip; 2 – flexible endoscope; 3 – handle; 4 – eye piece (or camera connector); 5 – light lead; 6 – light guide insertion

1.5.7 AIRWAY EXAMINATION

The primary objective of the airway examination is to assess the patient systematically. It will often form part of the oral-cavity/neck examination.

If the patient is in distress and there is any indication of an airway at risk, seek help immediately from an ENT senior and the anaesthetist on-call.

Airway pathology can arise due to a number of causes including trauma (severe maxillofacial injury, laryngeal injury, blast, burn or missile to face), infection (epiglottitis, supraglottitis, Ludwig's angina), physical obstruction (foreign body, soft tissue swelling of neck) and allergy (acute tongue and laryngeal oedema).

ESSENTIALS

Assessment and recognition of airway compromise

The following signs can indicate airway compromise:

- Position – tripod, orthopnea
- Skin colour
- Flaring of nares
- Pursed lips
- Drooling
- Accessory muscle use
- Altered mental status
- Inadequate rate or depth of ventilations, paradoxical chest movements
- Audible gasping, stridor or wheeze (Table 7).

Stertor	Stridor	
Snoring-like noise, typically originating from naso- or oropharyngeal obstruction	Noise due to upper airway obstruction	
Inspiratory, expiratory, or both	Supraglottic – inspiratory	
	Glottic – biphasic	
	Subglottic – biphasic	
	Tracheal – expiratory	

Table 7: Characterisation of stertor and stridor

Patients should be approached in an "ABCDE" manner. For further details on how to manage an airway emergency see section 2.1.

1.6 RADIOLOGY

Radiological investigations are often used in ENT to aid diagnosis, to monitor response to treatment, to help stage diseases such as cancer and for screening purposes. Imaging can also be used to guide surgical management by giving precise information regarding the pathology in relation to the surrounding anatomical structures.

As the junior doctor on-call, you may be asked to request imaging for patients. It is therefore worth keeping the following in mind:

- Radiological investigations should be used as an adjunct to a detailed history and clinical examination, and should not be used as a replacement.
- Give detailed information on the request form when asking for imaging – asking a question is often very useful and can guide the radiologist.
- If you are not sure whether you are requesting the correct type of scan, go and discuss this with the radiologist. Their advice is invaluable and may save the patient from having unnecessary or the wrong type of imaging done.
- Look at the scan yourself first to try and ascertain what the pathology might be – don't go straight to the report.

Some of the more common radiological investigations used are described below.

1.6.1 LATERAL SOFT TISSUE NECK X-RAY

Lateral soft tissue neck x-rays are useful when assessing ENT patients presenting with a number of symptoms ranging from dysphagia, foreign body ingestion and deep neck space infections such as retropharyngeal abscess.

ESSENTIALS

ESSENTIALS

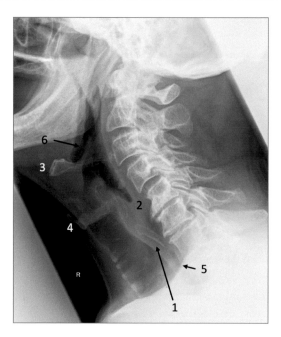

Figure 13: Lateral soft tissue neck x-ray: 1 – foreign body (chicken bone); 2 – pre vertebral soft tissue thickening; 3 – hyoid bone; 4 – thyroid cartilage; 5 – oesophageal air bubble (abnormal/sign of obstruction); 6 – epiglottis

An example of a lateral soft tissue neck x-ray is shown in Figure 13 with important structures labelled. The main steps in evaluating the x-ray are as follows:

- **Check adequacy of the x-ray:** neck should be held in extension and taken in inspiration. The film should include C7/T1 level of the spine.
- **Be aware of normal anatomy and common calcifications.**
- **Assess the bony contour:** a loss of cervical lordosis indicates pain and a possible obstruction.
- **Assess the thickness of the pre-vertebral soft tissues:**
  - o In adults, normal values for are less than 7 mm and less than 21 mm at C2/3 and C6/7 respectively;
  - o More often, a simple ratio in relation to the width of the vertebral body is used;
  - o Soft tissue widths greater than 30 % and 100 % of the upper and lower cervical vertebral bodies, respectively, are considered abnormal, and can represent inflammation secondary to a foreign body or infection;
  - o In children, normal values differ based on age.
- **Assess for air in the soft tissues:** this is indicative of a perforation or a gas-secreting anaerobic infection of the soft tissues.

- **Assess the cervical oesophagus:** an air-fluid level indicates an intraluminal obstruction.
- **Examine common foreign body sites:**
  - o The level of the cricopharyngeus should be reviewed, especially in the paediatric population (e.g. coin)
  - o Common sites for fish bones include the tonsils, tongue base, the valleculae and the piriform fossae; it should be kept in mind that many fish bones are not readily radio-opaque and cannot be ruled out on x-ray.

1.6.2 COMPUTED TOMOGRAPHY (CT) OF THE PARANASAL SINUSES

Computed tomography (CT) has become the radiologic modality of choice to assess the paranasal sinuses. Used in conjunction with careful history taking and examination including nasendoscopy, the sinus CT helps to establish disease extent and guide treatment. It is used not only as a diagnostic tool but as a key component in pre-operative surgical planning and as a roadmap intraoperatively when using navigation systems.

When interpreting sinus CTs, both axial and coronal cross-sections should be examined in a systematic manner, with bony and soft tissue windows used to evaluate the architecture of the bone and to look for the presence of disease.

Contrast-enhanced CTs are especially useful in evaluating vascular structures and soft tissue lesions including inflammatory and neoplastic pathology and may be used in conjunction with magnetic resonance imaging (MRI).

How to read a CT scan of the paranasal sinuses:

Examine coronal scans from front to back and axial scans from top to bottom.

The major structures to recognise are as follows and are shown in Figure 14.

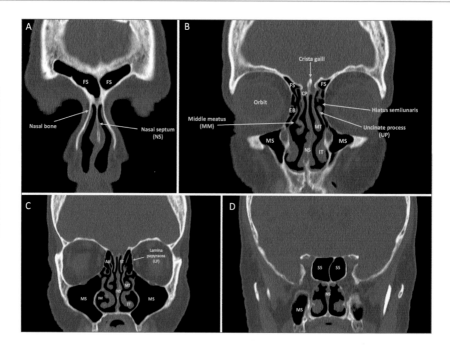

Figure 14: CT scan paranasal sinuses: A to D coronal sections anterior to posterior; FS – frontal sinus; NS – nasal septum; MS – maxillary sinus; EB – ethmoid bulla; CP – cribriform plate; IT – inferior turbinate; MT – middle turbinate; ST – superior turbinate; AE – anterior ethmoid air cells; SS – sphenoid sinus

Pre-operatively, there are key anatomic features that need to be reviewed on the CT scan to facilitate safe operating:

- Lamina papyracea – are there any dehiscences or bowing?
- Depth of the skull base/olfactory fossa – the Keros classification is used to classify the depth
- Location of the optic nerve and internal carotid artery in relation to the sphenoid sinus
- Position of the anterior ethmoid artery in relation to the skull base.

1.6.3 COMPUTED TOMOGRAPHY (CT) OF THE TEMPORAL BONE

A CT scan provides detailed information regarding the anatomy of the temporal bones and is the modality of choice when investigating pathology in this region. The temporal bone is made up of four bony segments (petrous, squamous, tympanic and mastoid) and houses multiple air spaces including the middle ear (tympanum) and mastoid cavity. (For further information regarding the anatomy of the middle ear and mastoid, see section 1.3.4.) Temporal bone CTs are useful for imaging middle ear and mastoid pathology, such as cholesteatoma, to assess the extent of disease and help with pre-operative surgical planning. The images are normally taken in axial and coronal planes (see Figure 15).

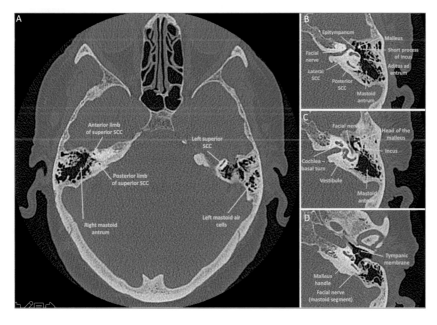

Figure 15: CT scan of temporal bone (axial view): A – whole scan view (bilateral temporal bones); B–D – axial sections superior to inferior of left temporal bone; SCC – semicircular canal

ESSENTIALS

1.7 AUDIOMETRY

Audiometry is a test used to measure the sensitivity and range of a person's hearing.

1.7.1 PURE-TONE AUDIOGRAM

This is a behavioural test designed to assess a patient's hearing using pure tones and allows assessment of both the central and peripheral auditory systems. The pure-tone thresholds give an indication of a patient's ability to hear the quietest audible sound at least 50 % of the time. An audiogram is a graphical representation of hearing sensitivity, with frequency plotted against intensity. Intensity is a measure of the sound power level measured in decibels hearing level (dBHL), which in turn is based on a standardised average derived from normal hearing individuals. Frequency is measured in hertz (Hz) and the range used for most audiograms is 250 to 8,000 Hz, as this correlates with speech frequencies.

Hearing loss can be described as mild, moderate, severe and profound and correlates with specific average hearing threshold levels (Table 8).

Hearing loss	Average hearing threshold levels (dBHL)
Mild	21–40
Moderate	41–70
Severe	71–90
Profound	>90

Table 8: Hearing loss and associated average hearing threshold levels

Hearing loss can also be classified as conductive, sensorineural or mixed. Conductive hearing loss (CHL) occurs secondary to abnormalities related to the external and middle ear. Examples of the former include complete wax occlusion, canal stenosis and atresias. Middle ear disease giving rise to conductive hearing deficits can be temporary and fluctuating (e.g. otitis media with effusion), or progressive (e.g. otosclerosis and cholesteatoma). CHL is typically represented by the presence of an air–bone gap on the audiogram of varying degrees of loss, which can be amenable to surgical intervention often with promising results (Figure 16C). Sensorineural hearing loss (SNHL) results from abnormalities of the cochlea, cochlear nerve or auditory pathway. These conditions may be hereditary or acquired and give rise to varying degrees of hearing deficits (Figure 16B). A combination of both conductive and SNHL components gives rise to a mixed type of loss. Both age-related hearing loss (presbycusis) and noise-induced hearing loss give characteristic patterns (figures 16D and 16E respectively).

ESSENTIALS

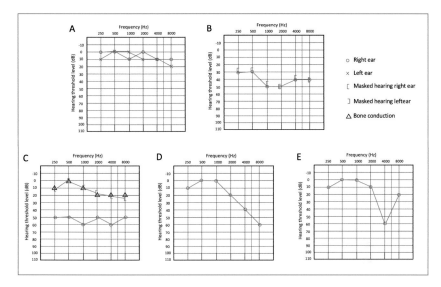

Figure 16: Audiograms with varying degrees of hearing loss: A – normal hearing; B – sensorineural hearing loss (SNHL); C – moderate conductive hearing loss; D – presbycusis; E – noise induced hearing loss

1.7.2 TYMPANOMETRY

Tympanometry is a test used to objectively measure tympanic membrane mobility and allows assessment of the middle ear status. The test is a measure of acoustic imittance and involves varying the pressure within the external ear whilst simultaneously exposing the ear to an acoustic tone. The reflected sound energy from the tympanic membrane is then measured. Middle ear pathology can result in stiffening of the tympanic membrane which in turn means more sound energy is reflected back. The results are represented graphically with three main types of tympanograms being produced according to the status of the tympanic membrane and middle ear. The canal volume is also routinely given on the test result.

Type A tympanogram

This indicates a normal peak and middle ear status. A Type A$_s$ tympanogram shows a shallower peak due to stiffening of the tympanic membrane (e.g. ossicular fixation). A Type A$_d$ tympanogram shows an abnormally high peak to the curve due to increased compliance (e.g. ossicular discontinuity or a flaccid tympanic membrane).

Type B tympanogram

A relatively flat trace in the presence of a normal canal volume can indicate the presence of middle ear effusion (e.g. otitis media with effusion). Where the canal volume is high, a flat trace represents the presence of a perforation or patent grommet in situ (typical canal volume for adults is 0.6–1.5 cm^3 and 0.4–1.0 cm^3 in children).

Type C tympanogram

This trace is indicated by a negative peak pressure and can represent the presence of Eustachian tube dysfunction and the presence of resolving or developing middle ear effusion.

Examples of common tympanometric traces are shown Figure 17.

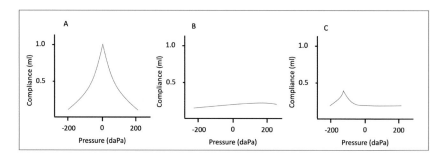

Figure 17: Tympanograms: A – Type A: normal; B – Type B: middle ear effusion or tympanic membrane perforation; C – Type C: middle ear negative pressure (usually secondary to Eustachian tube dysfunction)

1.8 ENT PRESCRIBING

This section introduces you to the common medications prescribed in ENT and serves as a quick guide to help you manage patients in the emergency and outpatient setting. Local guidelines may vary, therefore please check these before prescribing. In addition, certain medications in ENT are prescribed off-licence (especially in paediatrics).

1.8.1 EAR DROPS

Ear drops can generally be prescribed with the standard dosing (paediatric and adult):

- Three-to-four drops, three times a day for each ear in adults
- Standard course length is five-to-seven days, and should not be prescribed long term unless on specialist advice
- Length of each prescription should be tailored to the patient and pathology
- Prolonged or multiple courses of antibacterial drops can result in secondary fungal infections.

Antibiotic ear drops often leave a residue, which should not be mistaken for infection during examination. Commonly used preparations are detailed below (Table 9).

Medication	Dose/Preparations	Indications	Comments
Acetic acid	Strength: 2 % Standard dosing Preparation: EarCalm ®	Otitis externa – mild	Lower pH inhibits bacterial and fungal growth
Betametasone	Strength: 0.1 % Standard dosing Preparations: Betnesol®: betametasone 0.1 % Betnesol-N®: betametasone 0.1 %, neomycin 0.5 %	Otitis externa	Steroids to reduce inflammation Neomycin: aminoglycoside, has cochleotoxic properties * See note

ESSENTIALS

Medication	Dose/Preparations	Indications	Comments
Ciprofloxacin	Strength: 0.2 %, 0.3 % Standard dosing Preparations: Cetraxal®: ciprofloxacin 0.2 % Ciloxan®: ciprofloxacin 0.3 % Cilodex®: ciprofloxacin 0.3 %, dexamethasone	Otitis externa, acute otitis media	Not ototoxic Good pseudomonal cover
Gentamicin	Strength: 0.3 % Standard dosing Preparations: Genticin®: gentamicin 0.3 % Gentisone-HC®: gentamicin 0.3 %, hydrocortisone 1 %	Otitis externa, acute otitis media	Maximum 7 days and review Aminoglycoside – vestibulotoxic properties* Hydrocortisone: Steroid
Clotrimazole	Strength: 1 % solution Standard dosing Preparation: Canesten®	Fungal otitis externa	Use for a further 2 weeks once symptomatically and macroscopically clear of fungal infection
Clioquinol	Strength: 1 % Standard dosing Preparation: Locorten-Vioform®: flumetasone pivalate 0.02 %, clioquinol 1 %	Bacterial or fungal otitis externa Eczematous inflammation	Cloquinol: antibiotic, antifungal and antiprotozoal Flumetasone: steroid
Olive oil	No prescription limit	Impacted wax	Use for at least 1–2 weeks for good effect Softens the wax
Sodium bicarbonate	Sodium bicarbonate 5 % No prescription limit	Impacted wax	Use for at least 1–2 weeks for good effect Dissolves the wax

ESSENTIALS

Medication	Dose/Preparations	Indications	Comments
Other combination preparations:			
Otomize® spray	Neomycin sulfate 0.5 % Dexamethasone 0.1 % Acetic acid 2 % 1 spray three times/day	Otitis externa	*See note
Otosporin®	Hydrocortisone 1 % Neomycin sulphate Polymyxin B sulphate Standard dosing	Otitis externa	*See note
Sofradex®	Framycetin sulphate 0.5 % Dexamethasone 0.05 % Gramicidin 0.005 % Standard dosing	Otitis externa, acute otitis media	*See note
Triadcortyl Otocomb Otic® Tri-Adcortyl Otic®	Triamcinolone 0.1 % Neomycin 0.25 % Gramicidin 0.025 % Nystatin	Otitis externa	Instilled as cream via syringe to ear canal or coated on ribbon gauze as packing
Trimovate®	Clobetasone 0.05 % Oxytetracycline 3.0 % Nystatin	Otitis externa	Instilled as cream via syringe to ear canal or via ribbon gauze pack
BIPP – bismuth iodoform paraffin paste	Iodoform 40 % Bismuth 20 %	Antiseptic surgical packing	As paste for dressings or as impregnated ribbon gauze Can cause local hypersensitivity Avoid in patients with hyperthyroidism

Table 9: Common ear drops and their indication. *Note: Antibiotics may have ototoxic and vestibule-toxic effects; however, the topical application of drops is generally considered safe, especially in the presence of infection. Infection itself, if untreated, is potentially more toxic to the inner ear. Patients need to be counselled about this, to understand risk and how prescribing practice will vary in GP from ENT.

1.8.2 NASAL DROPS

Here we list common nasal prescriptions for a variety of pathologies that can be used in the acute or chronic setting (Table 10). Although we have provided dosing instructions, some nasal preparations can be used off-license (e.g. in the paediatric setting) on specialist advice.

Intranasal steroids have the best evidence base and are effective for the treatment of allergic rhinitis and chronic rhinosinusitis. The long-term use of intranasal steroids is safe (in both adult and paediatric populations) by selecting a low systemic bioavailability preparation and using the lowest dose to maintain therapeutic benefit.

Medication	Strength/Dose/Preparation	Indications	Comments
Antihistamines			
Azelastine hydrochloride	Rhinolast®: 0.1 % spray 1 spray each side, BD Licensed for age 6 and above	Allergic rhinitis	
Sodium cromoglicate	Strength: 2 % 1 spray each side, BD-QDS	Allergic rhinitis	
Steroids			
Betametasone	Betnesol® drops: 0.1 % 2–3 drops, BD-TDS Licensed age 6 and above Beconase® spray: 50 micrograms/spray 2 sprays each side, BD Licensed age 6 and above	Chronic rhinosinusitis (CRS), Rhinitis	Higher systemic bioavailability (44 %)

Medication	Strength/Dose/ Preparation	Indications	Comments
Fluticasone	Sprays: Avamys®: fluticasone furoate, 27.5 micrograms/spray Dose: 1–2 sprays each side, OD Licensed for age 6 and above Flixonase®: fluticsone proprionate, 50 micrograms/spray Dose: >12 years: 1–2 sprays each side, OD-BD Licensed for age 4 and above Nasule/drops: Flixonase®: fluticasone propionate, 400 micrograms/ampule (12 drops) Dose: ½ ampule (6 drops) each side, OD-BD	Chronic rhinosinusitis (CRS), allergic and non-allergic rhinitis	Systemic bioavailability: fluticasone furoate (0.5 %), fluticasone propionate (<1 %)
Mometasone furoate	50 micrograms/spray Dose: 1–2 sprays each side, OD-BD Nasonex® Licensed for age 3 and above	Chronic rhinosinusitis (CRS), allergic and non-allergic rhinitis	Systemic bioavailability (<0.1 %)
Dymista®	Fluticasone propionate and azelastine Dose: 1 spray each side, BD Licensed for age 12 and above	Allergic rhinitis, refractory non-allergic rhinitis	

ESSENTIALS

Medication	Strength/Dose/ Preparation	Indications	Comments
Others			
Ipratropium Bromide	Rinatec®: 21 micrograms/spray 2 sprays each side, BD-TDS	Vasomotor rhinitis	
Xylometazoline (Otrivine®)	Adult – 1 % (Drops/spray) 1 spray each side , OD-TDS PRN Paediatric 0.05 % (drops) 1–2 drops, OD-BD	Nasal decongestion: acute rhinosinusitis, pre-operatively for nasal surgery or during nasal examination	Short-term use only: adult – 7 days; paediatric – 5 days Prolonged and frequent use causes rhinitis medicamentosa

Table 10: Common nasal medication prescriptions and their indications

To improve delivery, minimise ingestion and improve compliance, it is important to instruct patients on how to deliver their nasal medications. When delivering nasal sprays, avoid contact with nasal septum by pointing nozzle towards the ear/turbinate (laterally). This will minimise side effects of epistaxis from contact and accidental trauma. When delivering nasal drops, lying supine with the patients head slightly off the end of the bed will allow the drops to coat the nasal cavity appropriately.

1.8.3 SALINE NASAL DOUCHING

Definition: The irrigation of nasal passages with saline solution, to clear debris and improve symptoms of obstruction.

Clinical uses:

1. Infection (e.g. chronic sinusitis)
2. Allergic rhinitis– prior to administering nasal medication, clearance of debris
3. Post-operative – clearing of nasal debris

Different types of nasal saline preparations are available over the counter in the form of sprays or solutions. Depending on the product, the resulting solution can be isotonic or hypertonic. Water alone is uncomfortable for the patient to irrigate with and often produces a stinging sensation. Patients can be advised to perform this two-to-three times a day.

Alternatively, patients can be advised to make their own preparation and buy a sinus rinse bottle over the counter. We provide here an example of how to prepare a saline douche mixture – your local trust will have an advice leaflet to give to patients with similar instructions.

Instructions:

1. Boil 500 ml of water
2. Add one teaspoon each of salt and bicarbonate of soda
3. Allow to cool to body temperature before use

1.8.4 ANTIBIOTICS

We provide here a guide for ENT antibiotic prescribing. Be aware that local microbiology guidelines can vary. Doses provided here (Table 11) are for standard adult dosing; paediatric prescribing varies by weight and age. Remember to also take into account co-morbid status (e.g. hepatic and renal impairment), interactions with other medications and side effects – these can be checked in a national approved formulary (e.g. the UK *British National Formulary (BNF)*).

Medication	Dose/Route	Indications	Comments
Penicillin V (phenoxymethyl-penicillin)	500 mg QDS/ Oral	Tonsillitis	Oral medication, not available IV
Benzylpenicillin	1.2 g QDS/IV	Tonsillitis	Oral switch is to penicillin V
Metronidazole	500 mg TDS/IV 400 mg TDS/ Oral	Deep neck space infections, suspected abscess formation (e.g. peritonsillar abscess, periorbital abscess)	Often added to another broad-spectrum antibiotic for additional anaerobic cover
Co-amoxiclav	1.2 g TDS/IV 375 mg, 625 mg/Oral	Acute sialoadenitis, acute mastoiditis, contaminated wounds	Good first-choice broad-spectrum antibiotic

ESSENTIALS

Medication	Dose/Route	Indications	Comments
Ciprofloxacin	400 mg BD-TDS/IV 500 mg BD/Oral	Severe otitis externa, necrotising otitis externa (NOE), pinna cellulitis	Has pseudomonal cover Can be given as high-dose oral route for NOE
Tazocin (tazobactam and piperacillin)	4.5 g TDS/IV	Necrotising otitis externa, aspiration pneumonia	Has pseudomonal cover
Flucloxacillin	400 mg QDS/Oral 1 g QDS/IV	Skin infections, cellulitis	Good staphylococcus cover
Ceftriaxone	2 g OD/IV	Complications of sinusitis, deep neck space infection, meningitis, sepsis	Often in combination with metronidazole for deep neck space infections or abscess
Cefuroxime	750 mg – 1.5 g QDS/IV 250 mg BD/PO	Sepsis, complications of sinusitis	

Table 11: Commonly used antibiotics in ENT and examples of typical conditions in which they are used

1.8.5 NASAL PACKING AND TOPICAL AGENTS

A number of agents are available for nasal packing and are described in Table 12 below. For insertion techniques, please see section 6.2.

Packing or topical agent	Description	Indications	Comments
Merocel®	Dry sponge tampon	Commonly available and cheap form of nasal pack, indicated in acute bleeds and post-operatively	Needs lubricating prior to insertion and inflating with sterile water once in place

ESSENTIALS

Packing or topical agent	Description	Indications	Comments
Rapid Rhino®	Balloon tampon	Acute epistaxis, including posterior bleeds (long or antero-posterior packs)	Remove the blue plastic encasing. Soak in sterile water for at least 30 seconds before insertion as this activates the carboxymethylcellulose coating that acts as a lubricant. Inflate with air after insertion.
Nasopore®	Dissolvable packing	Use for haemostasis for minimal bleeds by tamponade. Can reduce adhesions. Often used intraoperatively.	Transforms into an adhesive gel after 24–48 hours and then dissolves over the next fortnight
Bismuth iodoform paraffin paste (BIPP)	BIPP soaked onto ribbon gauze	Severe epistaxis, intraoperative packing or as an anterior pack after balloon/posterior pack insertion	Antimicrobial function of BIPP means that it can remain in situ for longer periods than other packs
Floseal® haemostatic matrix	Gelatin granules (bovine) and thrombin to form haemostatic liquid	Low flow bleeds or specific conditions not amenable to packing e.g. hereditary haemorrhagic telangiectasia (HHT)	Comes in a pack with applicator and mixing instructions to activate the matrix Aim to remove the clots before application to increase the chance of matrix reaching and covering the actual bleeding point

Table 12: Nasal packing and topical agents

1.8.6 HIGH-DOSE STEROID PRESCRIBING

Steroids are useful in ENT for their anti-inflammatory properties. All steroid dosing requires regular review and clear length of course (Table 13).

Avoid prolonged courses due to risk of adrenal suppression and gastric irritation. Wean doses depending on clinical condition and longer wean period for patients at risk of adrenal suppression due to a prolonged course (e.g. oral prednisolone course > 40 mg for over a week).

ESSENTIALS

Medication	Dose/Route	Indications	Comments
Dexamethasone	Dosing depending on indication and severity Oral (tablets/suspension) Available in 3.3 mg ampules (IV/Nebulised route)	Airway oedema Mucosal swelling	Adults: doses can vary depending on route and titrated to response Typical single from 4 mg – 10 mg or 4 mg TDS (for example, a single IV bolus of 6.6 mg can administered for emergencies) Paediatrics: *dose by weight and titrate to response Croup: 0.2 mg/kg Extubation cover: 0.3 mg/kg
Prednisolone	High-dose prescribing by weight 1 mg/kg (maximum of 60 mg)	Lower motor neuron facial nerve weakness (e.g. Bell's palsy, Ramsay Hunt syndrome), sudden unilateral sensorineural hearing loss, or step down from dexamethasone for airway oedema,	

Table 13: Indications and dosing of steroids in ENT conditions

1.8.7 NEBULISERS

Nebulisers can be used in the acute airway setting, as detailed in the emergencies chapter (see section 2.1) or for humidification (Table 14).

Medication	Dose	Indications	Comments
Adrenaline	Adrenaline 1 mg (1:1,000) delivered in a saline nebuliser	Airway oedema, at-risk airways, stridor	Can be given back to back in airway emergencies Titrate to response
Saline Nebuliser	0.9 % sodium chloride 5 ml ampules	For delivery of adrenaline nebuliser (e.g. 1 mg adrenaline diluted in 0.9 % sodium chloride made up to 5 ml) Airway humidification, to loosen airway secretions	Can be given back to back to humidify airway and prevent crusting – consider switching to humidified air/oxygen if frequent use required
Heliox (helium, oxygen)	According to oxygen requirement	Airway emergencies as temporising measure	Lower density and viscosity of helium–oxygen mixture make it easier to breathe in obstructive airway situations
Budesonide	Adult: 0.25–1 mg BD (max. 2 mg daily) Paediatric: 0.125–1 mg BD (max. 2 mg daily) Adjusted according to age and response	Airway oedema, stridor	Pulmicort® nebulised suspension not licensed for use for ages under 3 months

Table 14: Nebulisers used commonly in ENT

ESSENTIALS

CHAPTER 2: EMERGENCY DEPARTMENT

2.1 ACUTE AIRWAY COMPROMISE

This is an ENT emergency. You should contact your senior straight away. There will be experienced anaesthetists on site that can assist with any airway emergency if your senior is off-site and travelling in.

DEFINITION

Acute airway compromise is partial or total blockage of the airway. This can be caused by a number of different pathologies. Some common examples include:

- **Infective:** supraglottitis, epiglottitis, Ludwig's angina, parapharyngeal or retropharyngeal abscess
- **Inflammatory:** angioedema or anaphylaxis
- **Malignancy:** laryngeal mass
- **Trauma:** penetrating or blunt
- **Iatrogenic:** bilateral recurrent laryngeal nerve palsy following total thyroidectomy.

CLINICAL FEATURES

- **Stridor:**
  - o Inspiratory: point of obstruction most likely above the vocal cords
  - o Expiratory: point of obstruction most likely in the trachea
  - o Biphasic: point of obstruction most likely at the level of the vocal cords
- **Stertor:** Inspiratory noise induced by oropharyngeal obstruction

EXAMINATION

The patient should be assessed in resus. If the patient is in extremis, they may need to have their airway secured urgently. Examination should confirm the level of the obstruction. Ensure that you have a senior present prior to carrying out flexible nasendoscopy in case the patient loses their airway.

MANAGEMENT

- This should be completed using an Advanced Life Support (UK Resus Council) approach (ABCDE)
- Apply oxygen
- Give nebulised adrenaline (1 ml of 1:1000 adrenaline with 4 ml 0.9 % sodium chloride)
- Consider giving nebulised budesonide (1 mg budesonide ampule mixed with 4 ml of 0.9 % sodium chloride)
- Intravenous (IV) access and take bloods for FBC, U&Es, clotting and G&S, including blood cultures if pyrexial
- IV dexamethasone in order to reduce swelling (6.6 mg bolus in an adult)
- The Difficult Airway Society (DAS) provide guidance on how to manage a patient with a compromised/difficult airway (das.uk.com) – see Figure 18 and Figure 35
- In the case of a "can't intubate, can't oxygenate" scenario, guidance states that front of neck access using scalpel cricothyroidotomy should be performed (section 6.13)
- The patient's airway can then be formalised with a tracheostomy if required

FURTHER MANAGEMENT

Any further management depends on the cause of the airway compromise, but patients will often require a CT scan.

- o   Trauma: may need surgical exploration
- o   Infection: IV antibiotics/surgical drainage
- o   Malignancy: requires staging and MDT input

The patient is likely to need admission to HDU/ITU for further observation.

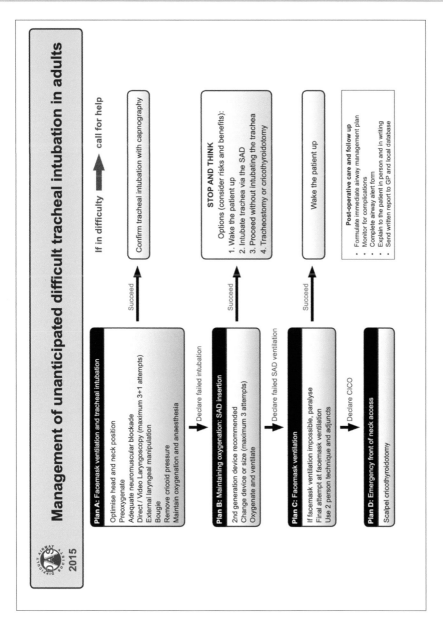

Figure 18: Management of the unanticipated difficult airway from the Difficult Airway Society

2.2 TONSILLITIS

DEFINITION

Tonsillitis is an acute infection of the tonsils. It can be either bacterial or viral. The most common causes are group B streptococcus, pneumococcus and *Haemophilus influenzae*.

CLINICAL FEATURES

- Odynophagia
- Dysphagia
- Pyrexia
- Halitosis
- Referred otalgia

EXAMINATION

Oral cavity: enlarged tonsils with patches of white exudate. The degree of enlargement can be classified in terms of the Brodsky grading system (Figure 19). The patient will most likely have enlarged anterior cervical lymph nodes.

Grade	Percentage of oropharynx occupied
1	≤25
2	26–50
3	51–75
4	>75

Figure 19: Brodsky tonsillar grading

MANAGEMENT

If not able to eat and drink, admit the patient. They will require:

- IV access
- FBC, U&Es, LFTs, glandular fever screen
- IV fluid resuscitation
- IV antibiotics – check with local guidelines but usually benzylpenicillin 1.2g QDS in adults
- Analgesia (both regular and break through)
- A bolus dose of dexamethasone 6.6 mg IV in an adult
- If glandular fever screen is positive, then advise the patient on refraining from alcohol especially if LFT deranged and on avoiding contact sports for at least six weeks due to potential abdominal organomegaly associated with glandular fever.

FURTHER MANAGEMENT

For those with recurrent tonsillitis, tonsillectomy may be the appropriate future course of action. Patients must meet the Scottish Intercollegiate Guidelines Network (SIGN) guidelines to meet the criteria for tonsillectomy which include:

- Sore throats that are due to tonsillitis
- Sore throats that are disabling and prevent normal functioning
- Frequency of episodes:
    - o Over seven episodes of tonsillitis in one year, or
    - o Five episodes per year for the two preceding years, or
    - o Three episodes per year for the three preceding years.

In addition to the SIGN guidelines, the Royal College of Surgeons' 2016 commissioning guide states that the following reasons are appropriate for tonsillectomy:

- Sleep disordered breathing in children less than 16 years
- Complications of tonsillitis such as quinsy.

EMERGENCY DEPARTMENT

2.3 QUINSY

DEFINITION

A quinsy or peritonsillar abscess is a complication of tonsillitis. It occurs when pus collects in the peritonsillar space and is caused by the same bacteria as tonsillitis. Early treatment is important to prevent extension to a parapharyngeal or retropharyngeal abscess.

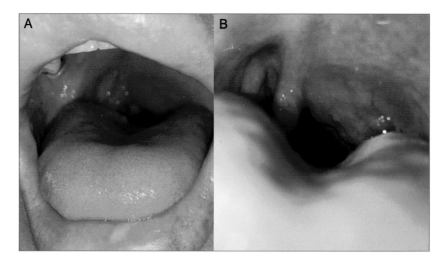

Figure 20: Left quinsy demonstrating asymmetry of palate, deviation of uvula and bulging peritonsillar area: A – external view; B – oropharynx

CLINICAL FEATURES

- Odynophagia
- Trismus
- Hot potato voice
- Pyrexia
- Halitosis
- Otalgia
- Peritonsillar swelling
- Uvula displacement away from the side of the quinsy

EMERGENCY DEPARTMENT

EXAMINATION

- Unilateral swelling in the oropharynx, medialising the tonsil (Figure 20)
- If there are concerns of parapharyngeal extension, suggested by hoarseness, stridor or dyspnoea, flexible nasendoscopy should be performed

MANAGEMENT

- IV access
- FBC, U&Es, LFTs
- IV fluid resuscitation
- IV antibiotics – check with local guidelines, usually benzylpenicillin 1.2 g QDS and metronidazole 500 mg TDS in adults
- Analgesia
- A bolus dose of IV dexamethasone, 6.6 mg IV in an adult
- Aspiration or incision and drainage of quinsy (see section 6.3)

FURTHER MANAGEMENT

- Quinsy patients should be offered tonsillectomy if they have had two or more episodes of quinsy or have had recurrent tonsillitis in the past.

EMERGENCY DEPARTMENT

2.4 EPIGLOTTITIS

This is an airway-threatening emergency so please involve your seniors immediately.

DEFINITION

Epiglottitis is an infection of the epiglottis that can potentially lead to airway compromise; you should involve your senior as soon as possible. It can be caused by bacterial, viral or fungal infections. In the past, *Haemophilus influenza* type b (Hib) was the most common cause; however, due to the Hib vaccination it has become rare, particularly in children.

CLINICAL FEATURES

- Hoarse voice
- Odynophagia
- Dysphagia
- Stridor
- Drooling
- Pyrexia

EXAMINATION

In an adult, flexible nasendoscopy should be performed to confirm diagnosis. In paediatric cases, if the patient is stridulous, this should be carried out in a safe environment such as the anaesthetic room or theatre, ensuring that the necessary team is present in case of airway compromise.

The epiglottis will appear swollen and erythematous as may the rest of the supraglottis. It may not be possible to see the vocal cords due to oedema.

EMERGENCY DEPARTMENT

MANAGEMENT

- IV access and fluid resuscitation
- FBC, U&Es, CRP, blood cultures
- IV antibiotics – check local guidelines
- Adrenaline nebulisers
- Budesonide nebuliser
- IV steroid bolus (IV dexamethasone 6.6 mg in adults or 150 micrograms/kg in children)
- If airway support is needed, the patient may need to go to ITU/HDU

FURTHER MANAGEMENT

- If the patient is intubated, they will require repeat nasendoscopy to monitor progress
- If the patient is not responding well to antibiotics, a neck CT scan with contrast is indicated to rule out a deep neck space infection or underlying malignancy.

EMERGENCY DEPARTMENT

2.5 NECK LUMP

DEFINITION

This is any lump or swelling within the neck. It can present acutely or gradually over time. The clinical history and the location of the neck lump can give you a lot of information about the likely cause. The differential diagnoses for a neck lump, depending on anatomical location, can be seen in Table 5. Causes are considered below in Table 15. It is important to assess the patient to exclude acute or impending airway compromise.

CLINICAL FEATURES

- Neck swelling
- Overlying skin changes
- Pain
- Fever
- Discharge

Red-flag symptoms:

- Dysphagia
- Dysphonia
- Weight loss
- B symptoms (fever, night sweats, weight loss)

EXAMINATION

- Neck examination to assess site, size, colour, tenderness, consistency and any tethering to the skin
- Movement of the lump with swallowing or tongue protrusion can assist in differentiating thyroglossal cysts from other lumps
- Examination of oral cavity and oropharynx for masses
- FNE to assess pharynx and larynx

MANAGEMENT

- This will depend on other examination findings and differential diagnoses
- Paediatrics: bloods for EBV, CMV, cat scratch fever – Bartonella henselae, TB (all causes of cervical lymphadenopathy)
- Adults: bloods for EBV, CMV, HIV, Lyme's disease, TB
- The patient will require imaging, which is usually USS +/- fine needle aspirate (FNA) to begin with; however, they may also require a CT or MRI for further assessment
- FNA cannot reliably detect lymphoma; a core biopsy or an open biopsy is required.

Category	Cause
Infective	Bacterial: tuberculosis, atypical mycobacteria, Bartonella henselae
	Viral: CMV, EBV, HIV
Inflammatory	Sjögren's syndrome, rheumatoid arthritis, sarcoid
Congenital	Thyroglossal duct cyst, dermoid cyst, lymphovascular malformation, branchial cleft cysts
Neoplasm	Benign: parotid gland (Warthin's tumour, pleomorphic adenoma), lipoma
	Malignant: primary/secondary, lymphoma
Endocrine	Thyroid nodules, thyroid goitre
Vascular	Carotid body tumour, subclavian artery aneurysm

Table 15: Types of neck lumps categorised by cause

FURTHER MANAGEMENT

- The neck lump may require excision for histology and microbiology if investigations are non-diagnostic.

2.6 OESOPHAGEAL FOREIGN BODY

DEFINITION

Oesophageal foreign bodies can be classed as soft or sharp. This can occur in the presence or absence of oesophageal pathology.

CLINICAL FEATURES

- Complete or partial dysphagia
- Unable to swallow secretions
- Pain when swallowing (often suggests a sharp object e.g. a chicken bone)
- History of choking
- Front or back chest pain (concern of perforation)

EXAMINATION

- Perform flexible nasendoscopy/laryngoscopy to rule out airway FB. Pooling of saliva in piriform fossa is seen if FB is high in oesophagus.
- Neck palpation to assess for surgical emphysema, which would indicate perforation.
- Level of obstruction as indicated by patient:
    - o Can help differentiate admission under ENT vs gastroenterology (low, non-sharp food bolus)
    - o Further to this, the time it takes for a sip of water to be regurgitated can help indicate the level of obstruction.

INVESTIGATION

- Lateral and AP soft tissue neck x-ray (Figure 13)
- Check previous history as it may hint at the possible level of obstruction (e.g. Barrett's oesophagus identified at a previous oesophago-gastro-duodenoscopy (OGD) or previous ENT review)

MANAGEMENT

- This is dependent on the local policies.
- Batteries: urgent emergency. This can lead to necrosis and perforation within two hours. The battery needs to be removed as early as possible.

EMERGENCY DEPARTMENT

- Soft foreign bodies:
  - o Admit the patient
  - o In many hospitals a patient with a low soft food bolus (below suprasternal notch) go to the gastroenterologists for OGD and removal of foreign body
  - o Trial IV hyoscine butylbromimde (Buscopan) (20 mg) +/- diazepam (5 mg)
  - o Trial of a fizzy drink
- Sharp foreign bodies:
  - o Managed by ENT
  - o Admit and keep NBM
  - o Involve registrar early; foreign body needs to be removed as soon as possible to prevent perforation
  - o Consent for rigid oesophagoscopy and removal of foreign body

Key timings: The risk of leaving a foreign body is oesophageal perforation. This is an immediate risk if the foreign body is a battery (aim to remove within two hours of impaction). Sharp foreign bodies should be removed within six hours and soft food boluses within 24 hours if they don't pass spontaneously.

FURTHER MANAGEMENT

If recurrent food boluses occur or there is a history of dysphagia, the patient will require a barium swallow as an outpatient and follow-up thereafter unless already undergone an OGD during the current admission. Battery ingestion can have late sequelae even after removal, so close monitoring (with serial imaging) is needed.

EMERGENCY DEPARTMENT

2.7 LUDWIG'S ANGINA

This is an airway-threatening emergency so please involve your seniors early.

DEFINITION

Infection in the floor of the mouth originating in the submandibular space, often secondary to a dental abscess. The swelling of the soft tissues causes elevation and posterior displacement of the tongue and can cause life-threatening airway obstruction.

CLINICAL FEATURES

- Recent dental abscess or submandibular gland infection
- Difficulty swallowing or breathing
- Immunocompromise or co-morbidities

EXAMINATION

- Floor of mouth swelling, crossing the midline, causing displacement of the tongue upwards and posteriorly
- Dental examination: tenderness to percussion, buccal mucosal swelling/abscess, state of dentition
- Trismus, voice change, increased work of breathing and signs of airway compromise
- Submandibular swelling and tenderness
- Sepsis

INVESTIGATION

- CT scan with contrast required to assess source of infection and abscess formation

MANAGEMENT

- Bloods to assess for infection – FBC, CRP, U&Es, blood cultures
- Broad-spectrum antibiotic cover (example: benzylpenicillin and metronidazole), appropriate resuscitation
- Steroids
- Intubation (recommend awake fibre-optic) if airway compromise or imminent compromise

EMERGENCY DEPARTMENT

- Bloods, including inflammatory markers
- CT with contrast if abscess formation suspected
- Incision and drainage under general anaesthetic if collection is present +/- extraction of teeth

FURTHER MANAGEMENT

If airway not secured with intubation or tracheostomy, very close observation is required, as there is a high mortality (from airway compromise) associated with Ludwig's angina. The origin source of the infection will need managing, too – for example, dental extraction by a maxillofacial surgeon.

EMERGENCY DEPARTMENT

2.8 ACUTE SIALADENITIS

DEFINITION

Infection of the salivary glands, usually viral or bacterial. Most cases occur in the parotid gland or submandibular glands.

CLINICAL FEATURES

- Pain, tenderness, erythema and warmth over the affected gland
- Can be bilateral or unilateral
- Usually caused by an obstructing stone (unilateral) or by hyposecretion of the gland (more commonly bilateral; more common in diabetic and dehydrated patients)
- Social and medical history in the elderly: note any deterioration in function; this may present as dehydration and resultant sialadenitis
- Past medical history including diabetes, Sjörgen's syndrome or autoimmune disease, or a history of anorexia; it can be seen in elderly inpatients not receiving adequate hydration

EXAMINATION

- Bilateral or unilateral
- Examine the other glands in head and neck
- Examine for the presence of palpable stones along the duct of the affected gland (usually bimanual palpation with one gloved hand in the patient's mouth)
- Assess hydration
- Check for blood glucose levels

MANAGEMENT

- Broad-spectrum antibiotics if bacterial. Increase fluid intake and apply good oral hygiene. Appropriate resuscitation if patient is septic. Use of sialagogues increases salivary production.
- Ultrasound scan if a stone or abscess is suspected. A parotid abscess is more likely in the presence of diabetes or immunosuppression.
- Involve the geriatricians in management of bilateral parotitis in the elderly – this is usually a symptom of a general decline in health or function as well as simple dehydration.

EMERGENCY
DEPARTMENT

- Viral aetiology includes mumps, coxsackievirus, herpes, influenza and parainfluenza. Confirmed mumps is a notifiable disease so Public Health England will need notifying if this is positive.

FURTHER MANAGEMENT

- Removal of the stone in the gland/duct can sometimes occur by massage, or alternatively by intra-oral incision, basket retrieval or extracorporeal shock wave lithotripsy.
- Occasionally in recurrent or chronic sialadenitis the gland may need excising.

EMERGENCY
DEPARTMENT

2.9 EPISTAXIS

DEFINITION

A nosebleed. Epistaxis is broadly categorised as a pathology of the nose or a problem with coagulation or hypertension.

CLINICAL FEATURES

- Flow: ongoing or stop/start
- Location of bleeding point: anteriorly in the nose or posteriorly (bleeding into the orophranyx)
- Right or left sided when started
- Preceding trauma
- History of nasal surgery
- Any systemic symptoms of blood loss: dizziness, shortness of breath or chest pain
- Past medical history, specifically hypertension, cardiovascular disease, anticoagulants or antiplatelet drugs, personal or familial coagulopathies, hereditary haemorrhagic telangiectasia (HHT). Make sure to ask about indication, dose, monitoring and most recent checks for anticoagulants.

EXAMINATION

- Examine the nasal cavity and oropharynx once the pressure has been applied for 10 minutes.
- Pack the patient's nose if they are in extremis but ideally proceed in a stepwise manner to stop the bleeding, as explained below.
- Auscultate the patient's chest and consider a CXR if any features of aspiration.

MANAGEMENT

- If the bleeding is not controlled with pressure, apply local anaesthetic with adrenaline to the septum.
- If the bleeding point is visible, apply silver nitrate cautery. Only apply this on one side as disrupting the perichondrial vasculature bilaterally can cause septal perforation.

- If this is not effective, then pack the nose. Use a nasal tampon, either a compressed sponge (e.g. Merocel®) or a balloon pack (Rapid Rhino®), or layered ribbon gauze coated in bismuth iodoform paraffin paste (BIPP). See section 6.2.
- If this is not adequately controlling the bleed, posterior packing will be required (section 6.2).
- Check the oropharynx again after each step to see if there is any ongoing bleeding.
- If on anti-platelets or anticoagulation, don't stop/reverse these if the bleeding is controlled by simple measures or anterior packs. Do reverse these if the bleeding is torrential or INR is high. For non-vitamin K antagonist oral anticoagulants (NOAC), call haematology for advice.
- Establish large bore intravenous access and send bloods: FBC, U&Es, G&S, clotting.
- Get an ECG if there is pre-existing cardiovascular disease.
- Recorded blood pressure (BP) at the time of admission may be reaction to the epistaxis rather than the cause of it.
- To establish the hypertension diagnosis, BP needs to be checked over a period of time (this is usually conducted in primary care; for any acute or inpatient advice consult the medical team).

FURTHER MANAGEMENT
- If the packs are in for over 24 hours, then start prophylactic antibiotics.
- The packs will be removed after a review by a senior colleague (normally on the ward round) – often the pressure from the packs will control the bleeding adequately enough to locate the bleeding point and cauterise it.
- If the bleeding is not controlled, further steps include topical haemostatic matrix application, surgery, angiography and others, depending on patient suitability.
- Before discharge, give the patient written epistaxis advice, including: don't blow the nose for two weeks, avoid hot food and strenuous activity for 48 hours, and apply antiseptic cream (e.g. Naseptin) to the nose twice a day for two weeks.
- Explain basic epistaxis first aid (nose pinch, ice pack application, wait, attend A&E if bleeding after 20 minutes) to the patient before discharge.

EMERGENCY DEPARTMENT

2.10 PERIORBITAL CELLULITIS

DEFINITION

Swelling around the orbit and the eyelid, secondary to an upper respiratory tract infection. Preseptal cellulitis means the infection is contained anterior to the orbital septum and it is often secondary to eyelid/lacrimal infection. Post-septal cellulitis refers to the infection posterior to the orbital septum and it is often secondary to sinus infection. The infection originates in the ethmoid or frontal sinuses and spreads via a dehiscent bony wall or emissary veins.

CLINICAL FEATURES

- Periorbital swelling, reduced vision, chemosis, proptosis, diplopia, ophthalmoplegia
- Colour vision is affected sooner than black and white; test the vision by checking colour identification.
- Headache; may suggest intra-cranial extension of infection
- Nasal discharge, sinus tenderness

EXAMINATION

- Eye examination: chemosis, proptosis, ability to open the eye, pupillary light reflex, eye movements
- Visual acuity assessment including colour vision using Ishihara plates
- Nasendoscopy: assess the nasal mucosa, middle meatus and take samples for microscopy, culture and sensitivity (MC&S) if pus apparent
- Cranial nerve (CN) examination

MANAGEMENT

- Bloods to assess for infection – FBC, CRP, U&Es, blood cultures
- Broad-spectrum antibiotics
- Nasal decongestant drops
- Nasal steroid medications
- Consider one-off dose of systemic steroid
- Intravenous fluids and analgesia

- CT scan: if central symptoms (drowsiness, fit, cranial nerve palsy, headache, vomiting), proptosis, ophthalmoplegia, deteriorating colour vision or acuity, bilateral periorbital oedema (cavernous sinus thrombosis), no improvement in 24–36 hours or swinging pyrexia >36 hours
- The results of the CT scan are classified according to Chandler's classification. A collection, unless a very small subperiosteal collection, needs surgical drainage, which can be done externally through a Lynch–Howarth incision or endoscopically.
- If the vision deteriorates rapidly then the eye may need to be decompressed urgently (with a lateral canthotomy then definitively with surgery).

FURTHER MANAGEMENT

If an abscess needs surgical drainage, a small drain may be placed externally. If performed endoscopically, a staged repeat procedure may be required. The visual symptoms and infective markers should improve post-operatively.

EMERGENCY
DEPARTMENT

2.11 ACUTE RHINOSINUSITIS

DEFINITION

Acute rhinosinusitis is acute inflammation and/or infection of the nasal cavity and paranasal sinuses.

CLINICAL FEATURES

- Nasal blockage, rhinorrhoea, hyposmia, facial pressure/pain, cacosmia, headache
- Fever
- Complications such as meningism, orbital cellulitis, Pott's puffy tumour

EXAMINATION

- Anterior rhinoscopy: purulent material in nasal cavity especially middle meatus (take a swab if pus present)
- Tender sinuses
- Assess visual acuity/colour vision/ophthalmoplegia if any periorbital swelling
- CN examination
- Examine teeth (exclude dental origin of infection)

MANAGEMENT

- Symptomatic care: five-day course nasal decongestant (e.g. Otrivine®), analgesia and nasal douching
- Topical nasal steroids
- Antibiotics if septic and consider antibiotics if symptoms persist over ten days or worsen after five days (penicillin or macrolide)
- If immunocompromised, significant co-morbidity or no response to the oral antibiotic treatment then admit for intravenous antibiotics (co-amoxiclav)
- If sinusitis complications or septic, admit for intravenous antibiotics and discuss with a senior colleague

FURTHER MANAGEMENT

If patient is getting more than three episodes a year, review in clinic and consider functional endoscopic sinus surgery (FESS). The EPOS (European Position Paper on Rhinosinusitis and Nasal Polyps) pocket guide details management of acute and chronic rhinosinusitis with and without polyps in adults and children.

2.12 FACIAL NERVE PALSY

DEFINITION

Facial nerve palsy is dysfunction of cranial nerve seven that causes facial weakness on the ipsilateral side. The diagnosis of a Bell's palsy (idiopathic) is a diagnosis of exclusion. The most important differentiator is to confirm that it is a lower motor neuron problem (upper motor neuron lesions are forehead sparing due to bilateral innervation). The most concerning cause of an (upper motor neuron) facial nerve palsy is a stroke, which needs immediate attention from the acute stroke/medical team, so always exclude this first.

CLINICAL FEATURES
- Time frame/onset (relevant to treatment)
- Hearing, auricular vesicles (indicates Ramsay Hunt syndrome), ear infection (can be secondary to this, especially if dehiscent facial nerve)
- Associated symptoms: any weakness elsewhere (relate to potential stroke or neurological problem)
- Preceding viral illness
- Paraesthesia/numbness (i.e. involvement of cranial nerve five)
- Exclude any associated head trauma (potential base of skull fracture)
- Past medical history: especially immunocompromise or diabetes

EXAMINATION
- Confirm lower motor neuron (no forehead sparing)
- Amount of weakness: grade according to the House–Brackmann score (Table 16)
- Ear: external ear/otoscopy vesicles, acute otitis media
- Parotid: any masses
- Complete cranial nerve examination

MANAGEMENT
- Diagnosis of exclusion – no investigations are necessary initially.
- Oral steroids if patient presents within 72 hours of onset – prednisolone 1 mg/kg up to 60 mg for seven days. Consider addition of an antiviral (evidence is equivocal).

EMERGENCY DEPARTMENT

- Lubricant eye drops during the day and eye ointment at night. Make sure the eye is protected/eyelids closed at night. Get urgent review if any eye irritation.
- Reassure patients about a good prognosis – 85 % recover, most within three-to-four months.

House–Brackmann Grading Scale	Degree of Movement	Description
I	Normal	Symmetrical function all areas
II	Slight	Slight weakness on close inspection
		Complete eye closure, minimal effort
III	Moderate	Weakness, not disfiguring, maybe not able to raise brow
		Complete eye closure on effort and asymmetrical mouth
		Obvious synkinesis
IV	Moderately severe	Obvious disfiguring weakness, unable to lift brow
		Incomplete eye closure, asymmetry of mouth even with maximal effort
		Severe synkinesis
V	Severe	Barely perceptible facial movements
VI	Total	No movement, loss of tone, no synkinesis or spasm

Table 16: House–Brackmann Grading Scale for facial nerve palsy. Grade the forehead, eye and mouth separately.

EMERGENCY DEPARTMENT

FURTHER MANAGEMENT

If patients do not recover by three months then arrange an MRI internal auditory meatus (IAMs). Consider referral to a specialist facial nerve clinic for further investigation and help with cosmesis or reanimation.

2.13 NASAL FOREIGN BODY

DEFINITION

Nasal foreign bodies are objects within the nasal cavity that should not normally be present. They are a common problem encountered in the emergency department amongst the paediatric population, especially under the age of five years. Common objects include beads, paper, pebbles, food, toys and button batteries. Longstanding nasal foreign bodies can form rhinoliths, which are hard calculi that result from the deposition of mineral salts.

CLINICAL FEATURES

- Unilateral nasal obstruction
- Unilateral foul-smelling discharge
- Epistaxis
- Unilateral vestibulitis
- Pain/discomfort

EXAMINATION

- Ensure good visualisation – use a headlight and a Thudichum nasal speculum. In paediatric group, you may be able to use an otoscope to perform anterior rhinoscopy.
- Suction may be required to remove mucopus.
- Foreign bodies are most commonly found either below the inferior turbinate or anterior to the middle turbinate.
- Organic foreign bodies such as food are more likely to cause irritation of the nasal mucosa compared to inorganic foreign bodies such as beads.
- Button batteries are especially dangerous, causing chemical burns, ulceration and liquefaction necrosis within the nose within hours of insertion, and must be removed urgently.
- Other foreign bodies, particularly non-organic objects such as beads and toys, do not require immediate removal; however, there remains a risk of potential airway aspiration.

MANAGEMENT

Preparation is key. A good headlight is essential as well as suitable instruments including a nasal speculum, Tilley nasal dressing forceps, suction and a wax hook. Multiple attempts may not be possible and should be avoided as they may cause mucosal trauma, posterior displacement of the foreign body with the risk of aspiration and unnecessary upset to the patient.

A cooperative patient is essential to allow examination and successful removal. For younger children, parents and other staff members may be needed to position/support the child and provide reassurance. Various techniques can be used to remove nasal foreign bodies, outlined in section 6.8.

FURTHER MANAGEMENT

- If the foreign body is successfully removed, both sides of the nose should be re-examined to ensure that there are no other foreign bodies present.
- In cases of failure to remove the foreign body, senior support should be requested.
- Where removal in clinic fails – the patient will need to be listed for examination under general anaesthetic and removal of the foreign body.
- In cases of infection, a short course of oral antibiotics such as co-amoxiclav should be prescribed.
- Routine follow-up is not required unless there is severe infection or trauma present.

EMERGENCY DEPARTMENT

2.14 EAR FOREIGN BODY

DEFINITION

Ear foreign bodies can be lodged within the ear canal or within the lobe or pinna (e.g. earrings). As in the case of nasal foreign bodies, children commonly present with foreign bodies within the ear canal such as beads, toys, seeds and pebbles. Adults may also present with foreign bodies in the ear canal such as insects, hearing aid inserts, ear plugs and cotton bud tips.

CLINICAL FEATURES

- Otalgia
- Irritation/buzzing noise
- Hearing loss
- Fullness in the ear
- Unilateral discharge
- Bleeding from the ear
- Asymptomatic

EXAMINATION

- Use an otoscope to examine the ear canal to ascertain the type and site of the foreign body.
- Examine both ears.
- In the case of foreign bodies within the lobe or pinna, use a headlight.

MANAGEMENT

- The key to successful removal of ear foreign bodies is good visualisation, having the appropriate equipment to hand and gaining the cooperation of the patient.
- For younger children, parents and other staff members may be needed to position/support the child and provide reassurance.
- Button batteries need to be removed urgently due to the risk of liquefaction necrosis and tympanic membrane perforation.
- Live insects need to be killed/immobilised prior to removal. Olive oil or lignocaine is used to for this.
- Earrings embedded in the ear lobe or helical rim can be explored and removed under local anaesthetic. If in doubt, contact a senior for advice.

- Good positioning of the patient is important – when using the microscope, ask the patient to lie on their back with their head supported by a pillow and turned away.

- If the object is very obvious in the lateral part of the ear canal, a headlight and aural speculum can be used with the patient sat upright.

- The first attempt at removal is usually the best, with success rates falling and the risk of complications such as trauma and bleeding increasing with further attempts. Further details can be found in section 6.8.

FURTHER MANAGEMENT

- After successful removal, examine the ear to check for any trauma and the state of the tympanic membrane.

- In the case of bleeding and infection, topical antibiotic ear drops may be indicated.

- In cases of uncomplicated foreign body removal, routine follow-up is not required.

- In cases of failure to remove the foreign body or in an uncooperative patient, seek senior advice and assistance. A general anaesthetic may be required.

EMERGENCY
DEPARTMENT

2.15 TYMPANIC MEMBRANE PERFORATION

DEFINITION

A hole or tear in the tympanic membrane (Figure 21). The main causes of tympanic membrane perforations are as follows:

- Infection e.g. acute suppurative otitis media
- Non-infective ear disease – cholesteatoma
- Trauma
    - o   Instrumentation (e.g. with cotton buds)
    - o   Sudden atmospheric overpressure (e.g. slap to the ear)
    - o   Excessive water pressure (e.g. scuba diving)
    - o   Head injury
    - o   Acid/welding burns
- Iatrogenic injury – inexpert aural irrigation/suction or residual perforation post-grommet insertion

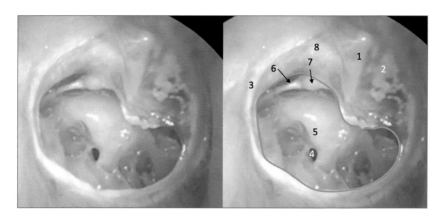

Figure 21: Tympanic membrane perforation (right side with labels overlaid): blue line – tympanic membrane perforation edge; 1 – handle of malleus; 2 – tympanosclerosis on the tympanic membrane; 3 – annulus; 4 – round window of cochlea; 5 – promontory of cochlea; 6 – stapedius tendon; 7 – stapes head; 8 – incus (behind tympanic membrane)

CLINICAL FEATURES

- Asymptomatic and seen incidentally on otoscopy
- Otalgia
- Otorrhoea – may be blood stained
- Hearing loss
- Tinnitus
- Dizziness
- Audible whistling during nose blowing/sneezing

EXAMINATION

- Otoscopic examination of both ears should be performed.
- The site and size of the perforation should be documented.
- Presence of active inflammation or discharge – a swab for microbiology should be taken if mucopus is present.
- If cholesteatoma is present with perforation, consider a CT temporal bone.
- In the case of head injury and potential skull fracture, a full otoneurological examination, including facial nerve assessment, should be undertaken. A CT scan should be performed.
- Audiometry and tympanometry should be performed.

MANAGEMENT

Conservative/medical management

- Dry traumatic perforations should be treated conservatively – patients should be advised to keep the ear dry. The majority of perforations will heal within three months.
- In the case of chronic dry perforations which are asymptomatic, no treatment is required. In the presence of symptomatic hearing loss, a hearing aid can be offered.
- Infection
  - o If there is evidence of infection, a swab should be taken and microsuction performed.
  - o Topical antibiotic ear drops should be prescribed.

EMERGENCY DEPARTMENT

o   Aminoglycoside-containing ear drops can used in patients with discharging ears in the presence of perforation (despite manufacturer warnings contra-indicating this, due to potential hearing damage). However, they should only be used in the presence of obvious infection and for no longer than two weeks, and the patient should be counselled about the potential risk.

o   Water precautions should be recommended.

- Cholesteatoma and perforation

    o   Perform microsuction (as tolerated by the patient).

    o   Treat active infection (as above). Pseudomonas is often the culprit.

    o   Refer for senior review.

- Temporal bone fractures

    o   See section 2.24.

Surgical management

- Surgical treatment of tympanic membrane perforations may be indicated in the following cases:

    o   Recurrent infections

    o   Conductive hearing loss

    o   Desire to swim/participate in water sports

    o   Hearing-aid users – use of hearing aids in the presence of perforation can predispose the user to recurrent infections.

- **Myringoplasty**

    o   This operation involves repairing the tympanic membrane using a graft without assessment of the ossicular chain.

    o   This graft material can include fat (fat plug myringoplasty), temporalis fascia, cartilage/perichondrium and synthetic biomaterials (e.g. Biodesign®).

    o   The ear can be operated on endoscopically or via a permeatal, endaural or postaural approach.

    o   In most cases, the tympanic membrane is elevated and the graft placed as an underlay.

- **Tympanoplasty**
  - o This operation involves grafting the tympanic membrane with assessment of the ossicular chain, with or without reconstruction of the ossicular chain where required.
  - o The ear can be approached as above and grafted using the various materials mentioned.

FURTHER MANAGEMENT

Patients should be followed up as appropriate:

- o Dry traumatic perforations – patients should be followed up in emergency clinic or with their GP.
- o Infection – patients should be seen in emergency clinic after an appropriate course of treatment to ensure resolution of symptoms.
- o Where there is any doubt, obtain advice from a senior.

EMERGENCY
DEPARTMENT

2.16 ACUTE OTITIS MEDIA

DEFINITION

Acute otitis media (AOM) is defined as the presence of middle ear inflammation with the presence of a mucopurulent effusion and associated systemic signs and symptoms of infection. Common causative organisms are listed in Table 17.

Bacterial	Viral
Streptococcus pneumoniae	Respiratory syncytial virus
Haemophilus influenzae	Influenza (A and B)
Moraxella catarrhalis	Adenovirus
Pseudomonas aeruginosa	Parainfluenza
Anaerobes e.g. *Bacteroides* species	Rhinovirus

Table 17: Common causative organisms in acute otitis media (bacterial and viral)

Risk factors for AOM include:

Host risk factors:

- Age <6 months
- Male sex
- Craniofacial abnormalities (e.g. cleft palate)
- Prematurity/low birth weight
- Immunodeficiency
- Recurrent URTI
- Gastro-oesophageal reflux
- Family history of otitis media

Environmental risk factors:

- Daycare/nursery attendance or multiple siblings (frequent contact with other children)
- Seasonal – increased in autumn and winter months
- Smoking/passive smoking
- Use of a dummy
- Formula feeding (breastfeeding offers protection)
- Prolonged bottle-feeding in the supine position

CLINICAL FEATURES

- Preceding URTI
- Otalgia – in younger children, often communicated by ear tugging/holding/rubbing
- Pyrexia
- Aural fullness
- Hearing loss
- Non-specific symptoms – poor feeding, irritability, behavioural change, crying, rhinorrhoea, cough, vomiting, diarrhoea, lethargy, febrile convulsions
- Relief from earache after noticing ear discharge (suggesting ear drum perforation with subsequent release of middle ear effusion and pressure)

EXAMINATION

- A general assessment of the patient should be made from the end of the bed:
    - o   Is the patient crying, restless, holding the ear?
    - o   Are they pyrexial? Note the observation chart.
- Otoscopy
    - o   Presence of a red/yellow/cloudy tympanic membrane
    - o   Bulging tympanic membrane with evidence of middle ear effusion
    - o   Perforation of the tympanic membrane with mucopurulent discharge
- Examination of the nose and throat should also be performed.

MANAGEMENT

- This is based on NICE guidance otitis media (acute): antimicrobial prescribing (Figure 22).
- AOM is a self-limiting condition in most cases, with symptoms lasting from three to seven days.
- Self-care is advised in all cases, including regular use of antipyretics/analgesics (e.g. paracetamol or ibuprofen).
- Evidence has shown that antibiotics make little difference to the number of children with AOM whose symptoms improve.

EMERGENCY
DEPARTMENT

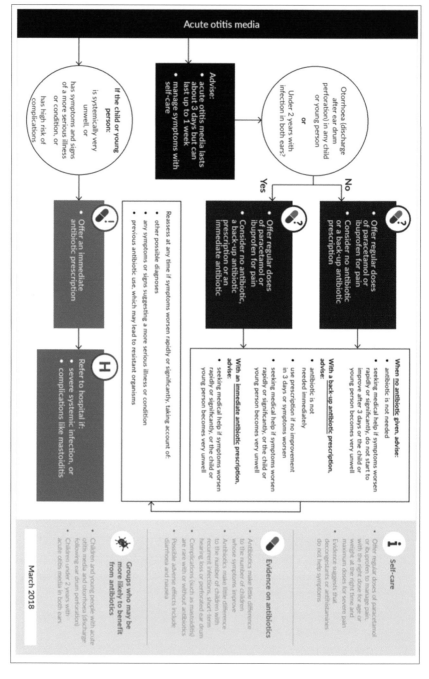

Figure 22: NICE antimicrobial prescribing in acute otitis media (2018)

- If an antibiotic is indicated, a five-to-seven day prescription should be prescribed (amoxicillin, or clarithromycin/erythromycin if the patient is allergic to penicillin).

- Often, patients presenting to hospital will already have been treated by the GP or be referred in with severe systemic infection or a suspected complication (see below). In these cases, a full history, examination and documentation of treatment to date should be made and patients should be managed in close conjunction with the paediatric team.

- In the case of severe systemic infection or a suspected complication, the case should be discussed with a senior. The patient will usually require the following:

  o IV access

  o Routine bloods (including CRP)

  o Blood cultures

  o Ear swab sent for microbiology, if discharge is present

  o IV antibiotics – co-amoxiclav is often used as first line (clarithromycin/erythromycin used in penicillin-allergic patients); however, local hospital prescribing guidelines should be checked and a discussion undertaken with microbiology as required.

  o Senior review will guide the need for further investigations (e.g. CT scan) and treatment.

FURTHER MANAGEMENT

- Complications of AOM include mastoiditis, intracranial sepsis and all of the complications of mastoiditis discussed in the next chapter. These will need to be treated accordingly – surgical intervention may be required as well as input from other subspecialty teams such as Neurosurgery.

- Routine follow up of uncomplicated cases of AOM is not required.

- In cases of recurrent AOM or chronic AOM, follow up in a consultant clinic will be required.

EMERGENCY DEPARTMENT

2.17 ACUTE MASTOIDITIS

DEFINITION

Inflammation which occurs in the mucosal lining of the mastoid air cells and antrum within the mastoid bone as a result of infection of the middle ear.

CLINICAL FEATURES

- Otalgia – in younger children, often communicated by restlessness and ear tugging/holding/rubbing
- Pyrexia
- Aural fullness
- Hearing loss
- Persistent pyrexia
- Pain deep in or behind the ear
- Non-specific symptoms – poor feeding, irritability, behavioural change, crying, rhinorrhoea, cough, vomiting, diarrhoea, lethargy, febrile convulsions
- Facial nerve palsy
- Central symptoms due to intracranial complications: e.g. headache, seizure

EXAMINATION

- Obliteration of postauricular skin crease
- Swelling and erythema over mastoid
- Tenderness over mastoid
- Forward protrusion of the pinna (if significant post-auricular swelling present due to oedema or abscess formation)
- Otoscopy
    - o Presence of a red/yellow/cloudy tympanic membrane
    - o Bulging tympanic membrane with evidence of middle ear effusion
    - o Perforation of the tympanic membrane with mucopurulent discharge
    - o Sagging of the posterosuperior meatal wall
- Swelling in the sternocleidomastoid/digastric/zygomatic regions (secondary to abscess formation)
- Facial nerve palsy

MANAGEMENT

Early diagnosis and treatment can prevent complications.

Patients will require the following:

- IV access
- Routine bloods (including CRP)
- Blood cultures
- Ear swab sent for microbiology, if discharge is present
- Urgent IV antibiotics – broad-spectrum antibiotics which penetrate the blood–brain barrier will be required. Hospital guidelines should be consulted, and microbiology advice should be sought.

    Imaging:

    - Most patients presenting with acute mastoiditis are diagnosed clinically.
    - CT/MRI scan of the brain and temporal bones should be used when suspecting intracranial complications.
    - Imaging may also be indicated when there is failure to improve or worsening of symptoms following 24 hours of treatment.
    - Imaging is also indicated in any case of neurological deficit.

    Surgical intervention:

    - The majority of patients with uncomplicated acute mastoiditis will improve with conservative management.
    - Failure to improve or a worsening of symptoms in 24 hours is an indication for operative intervention.
    - This may involve the following:
        - Incision and drainage of subperiosteal abscess
        - Cortical mastoidectomy
        - Myringotomy +/- grommet insertion.

EMERGENCY DEPARTMENT

COMPLICATIONS OF MASTOIDITIS

Temporal:

- Tympanic membrane perforation
- Facial nerve palsy
- Suppurative labyrinthitis (can cause dizziness)
- Labyrinthine fistula
- Petrositis (may give rise to Gradenigo syndrome – AOM, facial pain and abducens palsy)

Extratemporal

- Subperiosteal abscess (mastoid cortex)
- Bezold's abscess – abscess along upper part of sternocleidomastoid muscle
- Citelli's abscess – abscess along posterior belly of digastric muscle
- Luc's abscess – subperiosteal temporal/zygomatic abscess
- Carotid sheath abscess
- Para/retropharyngeal abscess

Intracranial

- Meningitis
- Lateral sinus thrombosis
- Brain abscess
- Otitic hydrocephalus
- Subdural empyema
- Cavernous sinus thrombosis

FURTHER MANAGEMENT

Patients with uncomplicated cases of acute mastoiditis treated successfully with IV antibiotics will be required to complete an oral course on discharge. They will normally be followed up in a consultant-led clinic.

Patients with complications secondary to acute mastoiditis will need to undergo treatment for that complication. For example, an intracranial abscess needs joint management with Neurosurgery.

2.18 OTITIS EXTERNA

DEFINITION

Otitis externa (OE) is defined as inflammation of the external auditory canal. Various forms exist:

- Diffuse OE – inflammation of external auditory canal, extending to the pinna and tympanic membrane
- Localised OE – folliculitis (infection of a hair follicle) within the ear canal which can progress to form a furuncle
- Necrotising OE – Extension of otitis externa beyond the ear canal into the surrounding bone. This is an aggressive form of OE that mainly occurs in the elderly, diabetic and immunocompromised population. It is also known as malignant otitis externa (see section 2.19).

CAUSES OF OTITIS EXTERNA

Acute

- Bacterial infection – the most common cause, with most infections caused by *Staphylococcus aureus* and *Pseudomonas aeruginosa*
- Fungal infection – causative organisms include *Candida albicans* and *Aspergillus* species.
- Dermatitis – seborrhoeic or contact (allergic/irritant)
- Trauma
- Environmental factors – e.g. water exposure

Chronic

- Dermatitis – seborrhoeic or contact (allergic/irritant)
- Fungal infection – secondary fungal infection due to prolonged use of antimicrobials/corticosteroids in the ear
- Bacterial infection – secondary to a persistent, low-grade infection, often as a result of unresolved/incompletely treated acute OE
- Chronic instrumentation (cleaning/scratching) causes trauma and loss of cerumen which in turn causes a low-grade inflammatory process within the ear canal. This leads to skin thickening and canal stenosis in the long term.

EMERGENCY DEPARTMENT

CLINICAL FEATURES

- Otalgia – can range from mild to severe deep-seated pain
- Aural fullness
- Hearing loss
- Tinnitus
- Itching
- Discharge from the ear – often malodourous
- Fever (not common)
- Pain on moving the pinna or opening or clenching the jaw
- History of water exposure – e.g. swimming/surfing
- History of preceding trauma to the ear canal – e.g. use of cotton buds

EXAMINATION

- Erythema and oedema of the external auditory canal +/- pinna
- Narrowing of the external auditory canal
- Eczematous changes affecting the ear canal/pinna
- Severe pain on traction of the pinna or pressure on the tragus
- Presence of discharge – serous/mucopurulent
- Fungal spores and hyphae may be present indicating fungal infection
- Cellulitis of the pinna (may extend beyond the ear to the neck)
- Difficulty visualising the tympanic membrane
- Inflammation of the tympanic membrane

MANAGEMENT

The key steps to treating otitis externa are:

1) Managing pain with the use of adequate analgesics
2) Microsuction to remove debris from the external ear canal
3) Administration of topical antibiotic/antifungal medications (insertion of an ear wick may be required to facilitate ear-drop application to the ear canal)
4) Avoidance of precipitating factors (e.g. water precautions, stopping instrumentation of the ear)
5) Furuncles should be incised and drained.

Acute Otitis Externa

- Take the key steps as outlined above:
    - o Give analgesics accordingly – regular paracetamol/NSAIDs. Codeine may be required.
    - o Perform microsuction – take care as it will be very tender (see section 6.7).
    - o Prescribe appropriate topical medication (see section 1.8.1).
    - o Give advice regarding self-care: water precautions, avoidance of instrumentation etc.
- If the external ear canal is very oedematous and narrowed, insert an ear wick.
    - o This is a dressing which acts as a sponge to help relieve the oedema and also acts to splint the ear canal open to allow the administered drops to pass to the site of infection. Inserted dry, they are inflated with antibiotic drops.
- If the patient has underlying skin conditions, ensure treatment is optimised (eczema) and allergens avoided (allergic dermatitis).
- Oral antibiotics:
    - o These are not indicated in the majority of cases.
    - o If the patient has evidence of cellulitis extending beyond the external ear canal but does not have extensive cellulitis and is systemically well, a seven-day course of oral antibiotics could be considered in addition to topical treatment.
    - o Can be considered in patients with immunocompromise/ diabetes mellitus (be aware of the potential for malignant otitis externa – see section 2.19).
- In the presence of spreading cellulitis, the patient should be admitted for IV antibiotics to treat the cellulitis in addition to topical treatment.
- If the patient has already had treatment for an acute OE and the symptoms are not improving:
    - o Check compliance with medication
    - o Ensure patients are undertaking the necessary self-care
    - o Consider whether or not a Pope wick is required
    - o Consider taking an ear swab for culture and sensitivities to guide further management.

EMERGENCY DEPARTMENT

Chronic Otitis Externa

- Treat as above.
- Fungal infections may be more prevalent due to prolonged or extensive use of topical antibiotics.
  - o Perform microsuction
  - o Prescribe a topical antifungal e.g. clotrimazole 1 % solution (Canesten®)
- Topical acetic acid (commercially available as EarCalm Spray) – application creates an acidic environment within the external auditory canal and impedes the growth of bacteria and fungi thus reducing the presence of infections.
- Topical corticosteroids, often in ointment form and combined with antibiotics/antifungals (e.g. Tri-adcortyl or Synalar-N), can also be instilled in the ear.

COMPLICATIONS

- Spreading cellulitis
- Abscess formation
- Myringitis
- Tympanic membrane perforation
- Fibrosis of the external ear canal leading to stenosis
- Necrotising otitis externa (see section 2.19)

FURTHER MANAGEMENT

- Patients should be followed up in emergency clinic for review.
- Pope wicks should be removed within 72 hours of insertion – the patient should be seen in clinic and reviewed.
- If symptoms are not resolving, consider why (see above).
- In patients with immunocompromise/diabetes mellitus with unresolving symptoms, be aware of the potential for necrotising otitis externa – see section 2.19.

2.19 NECROTISING OTITIS EXTERNA

DEFINITION

Necrotising otitis externa (NOE) is a severe infection of the external auditory canal and skull base. The infection begins as otitis externa that progresses into an osteomyelitis of the temporal bone. It most commonly affects patients who are diabetic, immunocompromised or elderly (or any combination thereof). It is also known as malignant otitis externa.

CLINICAL FEATURES

- Deep-seated and persistent otalgia
- Purulent otorrhoea
- Headaches
- History of diabetes or immunocompromise
- Hearing loss
- Vertigo
- Facial weakness, dysphagia, hoarseness – secondary to cranial nerve involvement

EXAMINATION

- Pain out of proportion to the findings on physical examination
- Granulation tissue in the floor of the external auditory canal at the osseocartilaginous junction – pathognomonic of NOE
- Exposed bone in external auditory canal
- Cranial nerve examination – may reveal facial palsy
- Signs of intracranial complications e.g. meningitis

INVESTIGATIONS

- Clinical history and examination will point to a diagnosis of NOE in most cases.
- ESR will be raised and acts as a useful indicator of response to treatment.
- Ear swabs/granulation tissue should be sent for microbiology – most commonly the causative organism is *Pseudomonas aeruginosa*.
- CT scan of the temporal bones will show evidence of osteomyelitis.
- MRI is also useful for evaluating soft tissue and for intracranial complications.

EMERGENCY DEPARTMENT

MANAGEMENT

- NOE carries a high rate of morbidity and mortality.
- Key steps in management are as follows:
  - o Microsuction of the ear
  - o Topical antibiotic drops (e.g. ciprofloxacin drops)
  - o Systemic antimicrobials (often long term i.e. 6–12 weeks)
  - o Strict diabetic control
  - o Diagnostic biopsy to exclude malignancy (one differential diagnosis is SCC)
  - o Treatment of underlying disorders giving rise to immunocompromise.
- Microbiology advice should be sought regarding the most appropriate systemic antibiotic. Often, a long course (12 weeks) is required. A common example is ciprofloxacin, as this has good pseudomonal cover.
- Hyperbaric oxygen can also be used as an adjunct in the treatment of NOE.
- Surgery may be indicated:
  - o Debridement of bony sequestrum
  - o Incision and drainage of abscess
  - o Facial nerve decompression.
- The presence of cranial nerve palsies suggests a poor prognosis:
  - o Facial nerve – eye care will be needed if patient is unable to close the eye
  - o Dysphagia – swallowing assessment will be required.

FURTHER MANAGEMENT

- Patients will need close monitoring.
- Treatment response will be indicated by an improvement in pain, falling ESR and CRP.
- Repeat CT scanning can be used to monitor treatment response but radiological appearances often lag behind.
- Radioisotope scans (e.g. Technetium Tc 99 methylene diphosphonate bone scanning) can be used as a more sensitive marker for treatment response.

2.20 ACUTE VERTIGO

DEFINITION

Vertigo is often described as the hallucination of movement. This is normally rotatory (i.e. the patient feels that the room is spinning or that they are spinning). Acute vertigo needs to be seen by the medical team first – there are many causes of acute dizziness, and none of the ENT causes are dangerous, whereas many of the medical conditions that cause acute dizziness are (including posterior circulatory stroke, myocardial infarction (MI), pulmonary embolism (PE) etc.).

CLINICAL FEATURES

- Nystagmus
- Nausea and vomiting
- Hearing loss
- Headache
- Recurrent episodes/first episode
- Length of episodes/persistent episode
- Other sensory disturbance (visual, proprioception etc.)

Figure 23 demonstrates a simple approach to vertigo. The patient history helps to narrow down the list of differentials in an area that can be intimidating due to its breadth and complexity. This does not replace the assessment by the medical team in an acute setting. Remember that good balance is contributed to by vision and proprioception as well as vestibular function, something particularly relevant for the more complicated, elderly or co-morbid patients. A dizzy clinic (or specialist falls clinic) referral can be very helpful in complex cases.

EMERGENCY DEPARTMENT

EMERGENCY
DEPARTMENT

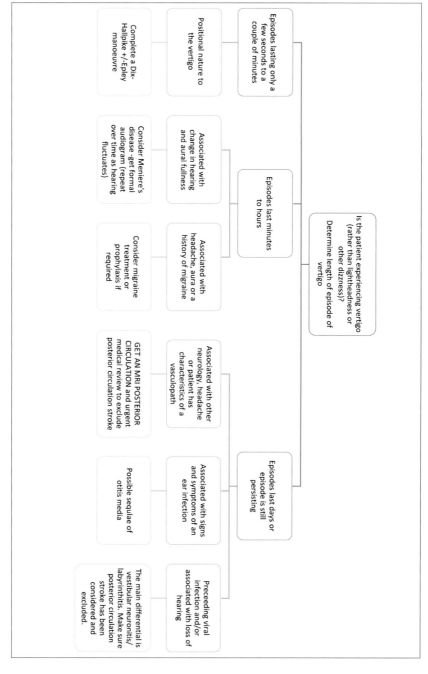

Figure 23: Management of vertigo, demonstrating the importance of the patient's history

EXAMINATION

- Ear examination
- Cranial nerve examination and examination for signs of central involvement or peripheral neuropathy
    - o   Upbeat or downbeat nystagmus is a red flag (central cause)
- Cerebellar signs – Romberg's and Unterberger's tests
- Dix–Hallpike test
- Hearing test

INVESTIGATIONS

- Most importantly with acute persistent vertigo, an MRI of the posterior circulation should be considered to exclude a stroke, especially if there are associated neurological signs and symptoms.

MANAGEMENT

- Due to the potential for serious underlying medical issues, dizzy patients should always be seen by medical teams acutely.
- Anti-emetics and vestibular sedatives (e.g. prochlorperazine) can be prescribed and admission may be required until the patient is safe to mobilise and eat and drink. This is normally under the care of the medical team.
- Advise the patient to contact the DVLA for assessment regarding fitness to drive.

FURTHER MANAGEMENT

- If the symptoms relate to a peripheral vestibular cause, the patients should be followed up in ENT consultant clinic, where a full history (length of episodes and associated symptoms) and a full examination are repeated. Vestibular function testing can be requested if necessary and/or vestibular rehabilitation.

EMERGENCY DEPARTMENT

2.21 SUDDEN ONSET HEARING LOSS

DEFINITION

Hearing loss occurring within 72 hours, which can be sensorineural or conductive in nature. Sudden sensorineural hearing loss can be considered an otologic emergency, and is defined as more than 30 dB hearing loss in three contiguous audiometric frequencies.

CLINICAL FEATURES

- Length of hearing loss
- Concurrent infection
- Trauma e.g. head injury
- Medications e.g. aspirin, some chemotherapeutic agents
- Previous sudden onset hearing loss
- Any associated symptoms

EXAMINATION

- External ear
- Otoscopy
- Cranial nerve examination
- Hearing test
- Tuning fork tests – is it conductive or sensorineural?
- Fistula test
- Romberg's test and Unteberger's test
- Assess gait

INVESTIGATIONS

- Full audiological assessment
    - o Pure-tone audiogram
    - o Tympanogram
- Bloods
    - o FBC and CRP – infection
    - o ESR, rheumatoid factor, ANA (autoimmune)
    - o INR and APTT – coagulopathy
    - o Fasting blood glucose (diabetes mellitus)
    - o Lipid screen (hyperlipidaemia)

- Imaging
    - o   MRI [cerebellopontine angle (CPA) lesions]
    - o   CT temporal bones (trauma)

MANAGEMENT

- High-dose steroids (prednisolone 1 mg/kg up to 60 mg for 7 days) if sensorineural hearing loss with onset within 72 hours. Consider gastric protection.
- If conductive hearing loss, acute treatment is not required but investigation into the cause should be done by a full history/ examination/imaging.
- If bilateral or only hearing ear, consider urgent management (treatment and investigation) including oral/intratympanic steroids.

FURTHER MANAGEMENT

- Hearing assessment in a consultant clinic and consideration of hearing aid. If there is unilateral hearing loss with asymmetry of 15 dB or more at any two adjacent frequencies (between 0.5 and 8 kHz) investigate with an MRI of internal auditory meati (IAMs).

EMERGENCY DEPARTMENT

2.22 PERICHONDRITIS

DEFINITION

Inflammation of the perichondrium (the connective tissue layer surrounding the pinna cartilage).

CLINICAL FEATURES

- Painful swelling and warmth of the pinna
- Preceding otitis externa, foreign body insertion or trauma

EXAMINATION

- Erythema, warmth, tenderness and swelling over the pinna cartilage
- Exclude collection (will need surgical drainage)
- Examine external ear canal and tympanic membrane – there may also be associated otitis externa

INVESTIGATIONS

- Microscopy, culture and sensitivity (MC&S) swab can be taken if there is otitis externa with discharge, or a pinna collection. The underlying microbiology is often pseudomonas aeruginosa.

MANAGEMENT

- This needs aggressive treatment to avoid chondritis and progression to chondral collapse (causing deformity or a "cauliflower ear"). Ciprofloxacin has good cartilage penetration.
- Remove any foreign bodies such as earrings
- Incision and drainage if there is a fluid collection/abscess
- If patients present repeatedly, consider relapsing polychondritis.

2.23 FACIAL TRAUMA AND HEAD INJURIES

DEFINITION

Head injury patients with a septal haematoma, pinna haematoma or laceration to the pinna or nose are often referred to ENT from A&E. Temporal bone fractures are discussed in the section below. It is important to be sure that the patient has had a severe head injury excluded before focussing on the ENT problem.

Septal haematoma

A septal haematoma is a collection of blood between the nasal septal cartilage and the perichondrium. Its presence causes a large red boggy swelling of the septum which can be bilateral. The haematoma disrupts the blood supply to the septum, meaning there is a risk of avascular necrosis of the cartilage if not treated promptly (within 24 hours).

Nasal fractures

Nasal fractures need to be seen in ENT emergency clinic at about five-to-seven days after injury. This allows time for oedema to settle down and assessment of asymmetry can be made. If there is bone displacement with the nasal fracture, this may need a manipulation under anaesthesia (section 6.12), which needs to be performed within two weeks of injury, while the bony fusion is still soft/not fully healed. This can be done under local or general anaesthesia. When patients are referred with a nasal fracture, it is important to make sure the assessing clinician has excluded a septal haematoma and assessed the severity of the head injury. Detailed documentation of the findings (ideally with photographs) is paramount as nasal fracture cases may involve the police and the court in future.

Pinna haematoma

A pinna haematoma is a collection of blood between the pinna cartilage and the perichondrium, and the same risk of cartilage damage if left untreated applies.

Lacerations

Lacerations to the pinna and nose are managed similarly: the wound needs to be cleaned, cartilage reapproximated (if there is excess cartilage due to skin loss in the ear, this can be trimmed) and the skin closed over this, with oral antibiotic cover given.

EMERGENCY DEPARTMENT

CLINICAL FEATURES

- Both nasal septal and pinna haematomas are painful
- History of preceding trauma
- Note any anticoagulation or antiplatelet therapy
- Other injuries and head injury symptoms

EXAMINATION

- Nasal septal haematoma: often bilateral boggy swelling, erythema, nasal obstruction, tender, epistaxis
- Nasal fracture: degree of asymmetry/displacement, exclude septal haematoma
- Pinna haematoma: fluctuant swelling in pinna
- Lacerations: assess location, extent, cartilage involvement and any skin loss
- Assess for head injury and injury to other facial structures if not already completed

MANAGEMENT

- Make sure patients are managed according to Advanced Trauma Life Support (ATLS) principles, with life-threatening injuries managed appropriately first.
- Occasionally, patients with septal haematomas will have ongoing epistaxis and need nasal packing. It would be appropriate to aspirate or drain these under local anaesthetic and then pack the nose; the haematoma can be reassessed when the packs are removed. Make sure this is documented and handed over.
- The principles of incision and drainage of haematomas, and laceration closure, are explored further in Chapter 6: Procedures.

FURTHER MANAGEMENT

No further management is usually necessary, unless a patient has significant skin loss around a laceration site. If this is the case, then input from a facial plastics specialist will usually be required for reconstruction; however, this does not need to be arranged in the acute setting.

2.24 TEMPORAL BONE FRACTURE

DEFINITION

This is a serious head injury and should be managed accordingly. A fracture through the temporal bone can be associated with hearing loss, facial nerve damage and vertigo, especially if the fracture involves the otic capsule. Patients may be referred while in ITU and assessment may initially be limited.

CLINICAL FEATURES

- Head injury: any loss of consciousness, change in vision, vomiting
- Facial weakness – onset and severity
- Hearing loss, vestibular dysfunction
- Clear nasal or ear discharge (suggesting possible cerebrospinal fluid (CSF) rhinorrhoea)

EXAMINATION

- External auditory canal laceration, haemotympanum or tympanic membrane perforation
- Mastoid haematoma/bruising (Battle's sign) or periorbital bruising
- Facial paralysis (House–Brackmann score – Table 16)
- Cranial nerve examination
- Hearing loss
- Vestibular dysfunction
- CSF leakage

INVESTIGATIONS

- High-resolution CT temporal bone
  - o Longitudinal fracture (70–80 %) associated with conductive hearing loss
  - o Transverse fracture (10–20 %) associated with SNHL
  - o Most are likely to be a mixed picture – most important is breach of otic capsule, which makes SNHL and facial nerve weakness more likely
- Pure-tone audiogram

EMERGENCY DEPARTMENT

MANAGEMENT

- Manage head injury
- Document any facial nerve injury and get audiological assessment
- Document any CSF leak – will likely need to be an inpatient due to increased meningitis risk while a leak is ongoing. A lumbar drain or occasionally surgical repair will be required.
- For a delayed onset facial nerve palsy, start high-dose steroids – the delayed onset indicates the nerve was intact after the injury and therefore the paralysis is likely to be secondary to compression due to oedema which may be relieved by steroids (Table 13).

FURTHER MANAGEMENT

- If the patient is stable and has a House–Brackmann VI facial nerve palsy, electroneuronography (ENOG) can be used to investigate nerve integrity and conduction. With a worse than 90 % ENOG at 30 days, the facial nerve should be decompressed surgically. Other management of facial nerve palsies can be found in section 2.12.

2.25 PENETRATING NECK TRAUMA

DEFINITION

Any sharp injury to the neck where the skin has been breached. A breach of the platysma muscle will need further investigation: this can be surgical or with imaging. There may be other injuries, so cases should be managed according to ATLS principles.

CLINICAL FEATURES

- History of trauma and nature of injury including instrument causing injury
- Extent of haemorrhage from wound site
- Extent of haematoma and resultant compression of vital organs
- Stridor, dysphonia, dyspnoea, haemoptysis
- Complete dysphagia

EXAMINATION

- Assess whether the injury breaches the platysma muscle
- Location of the injury
- Haemorrhage from the wound site, air bubbling from the wound
- Signs suggesting potential or impending airway compromise: stridor, dysphonia, dyspnoea, haemoptysis
- Neurological deficits
- Flexible nasendoscopy: mucosal tears, haemorrhage, oedema, pooling of saliva, airway compromise
- Document wound characteristics (e.g. site, size, pattern, location); the information may be required for police investigations and medicolegal reasons in future
- Check for any coagulopathies or anticoagulants

INVESTIGATIONS AND MANAGEMENT

- If the patient has "hard signs" of shock, expanding haematoma, audible bruit/palpable thrill, airway compromise, wound bubbling, subcutaneous emphysema, stridor, hoarseness, odynophagia or neurological deficit, proceed straight to theatre for stabilisation of the airway and wound exploration, plus or minus pharyngo-oesophagoscopy.

EMERGENCY DEPARTMENT

- If stable, high-resolution computed tomography with angiography should be performed. This may indicate neck exploration in theatre is required.

FURTHER MANAGEMENT

- Barium swallow to be done once patient is stable (if an oesophageal tear is suspected; to evaluate healing).

EMERGENCY
DEPARTMENT

2.26 BLUNT NECK TRAUMA

DEFINITION

Non-penetrative trauma to the neck. This can cause spinal injuries, but also laryngotracheal injury and pharyngo-oesophageal injury. Strangulation injuries (such as assault or attempted hanging) can cause thyroid cartilage fractures and hyoid fractures. Hyperextension injuries are more likely to cause tracheal tears, laryngeal fractures or even laryngotracheal separation. There may be airway compromise, a cervical spine fracture and other injuries so manage the case according to ATLS principles.

CLINICAL FEATURES

- History of trauma
- Dysphonia
- Haemoptysis
- Complete dysphagia

EXAMINATION

- Airway compromise
- Drooling
- Flexible nasendoscopy: mucosal tears, haemorrhage, oedema, pooling of saliva, airway compromise
- Surgical emphysema of the neck, bruising and tenderness

INVESTIGATIONS

- CT +/- angiography of neck if patient is stable to assess for laryngeal fractures, vascular injury and/or oesophageal tears
- Pharyngoscopy and oeosphagoscopy to assess injury if indicated (as requires general anaesthetic)

MANAGEMENT

- Secure patient's airway if compromised or impending compromise with early intubation.
- Some laryngeal fractures will require fixation; this will need to be discussed with a tertiary centre that performs these after stabilisation of the patient's airway, CT scan and assessment/stabilisation of any other injuries.

- Place the patient nil by mouth (NBM) if confirmed or suspected pharyngeal/oesophageal tear. The patient will need a fluoroscopically guided nasogastric (NG) tube placed for feeding when stable. Sometimes a tear over two centimetres will need to be closed surgically.

FURTHER MANAGEMENT

- Gastrograffin swallow should be performed once the patient is stable, if an oesophageal tear is suspected. This should be followed by staged barium swallow tests (to evaluate healing).

CHAPTER 3: OPERATING THEATRE

3.1 GENERAL PRINCIPLES

In the UK, surgical cases are classified according to the categories outlined by the National Confidential Enquiry into Patient Outcome and Death (NCEPOD) (Table 18). This classification helps clinicians triage and manage theatre time according to the urgency of each case. In an emergency, it will usually be the responsibility of your on-call senior to assign the NCEPOD category; however, all members of the team should be familiar with this in order to support the perioperative management of the patient.

Code	Category	Description	Target Time to Theatre	Expected Location	Examples
1	Immediate	Immediate (A) lifesaving or (B) limb- or organ-saving intervention. Resuscitation simultaneous with surgical treatment	Within minutes of decision to operate	Next available operating theatre – "break-in" to existing lists if required	Airway obstruction – intubation +/- tracheostomy. Arrest of bleeding (e.g. post-tonsillectomy bleed, expanding neck haematoma with airway distress)
2	Urgent	Acute onset or deterioration of conditions that threaten life, limb or organ survival; fixation of fractures; relief of distressing symptoms	Within hours of decision to operate and normally once resuscitation completed	Day-time "emergency" list or out-of-hours emergency theatre (including at night)	Foreign body removal from upper aerodigestive tract (e.g. battery, sharp foreign body). Drainage of abscess (e.g. periorbital abscess, mastoid abscess). Drainage of haematoma (e.g. septal haematoma)

Code	Category	Description	Target Time to Theatre	Expected Location	Examples
3	Expedited	Stable patient requiring early intervention for a condition that is not an immediate threat to life, limb or organ survival	Within days of decision to operate	Elective list which has "spare" capacity or day-time "emergency" list (not at night)	Excision/ debulking of tumours with potential to bleed or obstruct
4	Elective	Surgical procedure planned or booked in advance of routine admission to hospital	Planned	Elective theatre list booked and planned prior to admission	Manipulation of nasal fracture (selected cases) Removal of inorganic foreign body from ear (non-battery)

Table 18: NCEPOD Surgery Classification Adapted with Examples of ENT Emergencies

See: www.ncepod.org.uk/classification.html

OPERATING THEATRE

3.2 SPECIALIST THEATRE EQUIPMENT

The wide range of specialist equipment and procedures across the different subspecialties of ENT may be unfamiliar to the junior doctor. This section will serve as a general overview to familiarise you with the different surgical approaches and equipment you may learn to use through your ENT placement. When considering theatre set up and positioning, a major difference in ENT is that the surgeon and anaesthetist are both working at the head-end of the patient, and airway procedures with a "shared-airway" (such as laryngobronchoscopy or tracheostomy) will require good communication and teamwork between all involved.

3.2.1 ENDOSCOPIC SURGERY

Endoscopic surgery is used in sinonasal surgery, anterior skull base surgery, airway surgery and increasingly in ear surgery, for both visualisation of the operative field and documentation of findings. Most commonly used is a 0° endoscope but other angulations are available depending on the access and visual field required.

In addition to the endoscopic stack and screens, additional equipment may be required for the same procedure, such as micro-debriders, drills and navigation systems. Therefore, the arrangement of equipment, patient position and positions of the anaesthetic machine, scrub table and operating surgeon requires pre-operative planning to establish the most ergonomic position for operating.

Examples: functional endoscopic sinus surgery (FESS), airway and upper aerodigestive tract assessment (e.g. microlaryngoscopy, laryngotracheobronchoscopy, airway foreign body removal), middle ear surgery (e.g. cholesteatoma surgery, tympanoplasty)

Key points:
- Ensure that you use the right size/length and type of scope for the procedure
- Check that images are in focus and white-balanced for accurate visualisation

3.2.2 SURGICAL MICROSCOPE

The most common procedure performed under the microscope in ENT is microsuction of the ear in clinic (section 6.7). Operating microscopes have more features than their clinic counterparts such as focal length

OPERATING THEATRE

adjustment. Sterile drapes are available to keep the microscope arm and eyepieces sterile for procedures such as middle ear surgery.

The general principles of setting up a microscope apply to both the clinic and operative microscope.

Key points:

- Know your inter-pupillary distance (IPD) and adjust this for the eyepiece at the start of the procedure.
- Check the balance of the microscope, such that you can easily change the position and angle during the procedure.
- Familiarise yourself with the zoom and focus buttons/knobs.
- Check that the working distance for the objective lens on the microscope is appropriate for the procedure and equipment (general rule: Laryngeal surgery – 400 mm; ear surgery – 250 mm).

Examples: middle ear surgery (e.g. cholesteatoma surgery, cochlear implant, ossiculoplasty, tympanoplasty)

3.2.3 NERVE MONITORS

Nerve monitors are electromyographic (EMG) monitors used to measure any change in function of a nerve during an operation by measuring muscle tone (of the relevant/related muscle). A common example is that of the facial nerve. This is monitored during middle ear surgery by electrodes placed in the temporalis muscle and orbicularis oris muscle to measure functional output of two branches of the facial nerve (more branch monitoring can be added in parotid surgery). Stimulation probes can be added to be used intraoperatively to stimulate nerve function, monitored by a response through the EMG.

Examples: Facial nerve monitoring, recurrent laryngeal nerve monitoring, acoustic monitoring

Key Points:

- Get a senior to demonstrate how to apply the monitor
- Make sure to check the monitor check points and function before scrubbing

3.2.4 LASERS

As an ENT junior you are unlikely to be operating lasers used in certain subspecialty operations. Nevertheless, you may be present in theatre and you need to be aware of the relevant safety aspects paramount to avoid injury to the patient and theatre staff.

Examples: laryngeal laser surgery, trans-oral laser surgery, stapedectomy and middle ear surgery

Benefits of laser:

- Has properties of cutting, coagulation, haemostasis and vaporisation of tissue
- Precision leads to minimal bleeding and trauma
- Different delivery systems – useful for areas of difficult access and minimally invasive surgery

Risks:

- Fire (including airway fire in the patient)
- Injury to the patient
- Injury to staff

Precautions:

- Theatre environment must be laser-safe (windows covered, warning signs displayed, theatre doors locked and movement in and out of the operating theatre restricted to avoid breach of laser-safety conditions)
- Only adequately trained personnel should operate a laser and the associated equipment
- Eye protection is required for the patient and all personnel present
- Flammable equipment, medical gases and other materials should be removed
- Laser-safe endotracheal tubes must be used for GA

Dry materials in the operating field should be soaked in saline and a syringe of saline on standby for use in an emergency airway fire (rare).

OPERATING THEATRE

3.3 CONSENTING PATIENTS FOR THEATRE

3.3.1 CONSENTING PATIENTS

For the process of obtaining consent the patient is required to make an informed decision based on information provided by the clinician. In accordance with the Mental Capacity Act 2005, for a patient to give consent he or she must be able to:

- Understand the information being given
- Retain the information
- Weigh up the pros and cons
- Communicate his or her decision.

Consent should be taken by the surgeon carrying out the procedure, or a member of their team who has adequate knowledge of the procedure, the benefits and the potential risks.

In the elective setting the patient should be consented in clinic, allowing time for them to reflect on the procedure. They should also be provided with extra information in the form of leaflets or websites. On the day of surgery, consent is confirmed with the patient and this is documented on the consent form. In the emergency setting, time is of the essence and therefore the patient is often consented in the emergency department or on the ward.

As per the Royal College of Surgeons' 'Good Surgical Practice' guidelines (2014), a discussion around taking consent should cover the following:

- The patient's diagnosis and prognosis
- Options for treatment, including non-operative care and no treatment
- The purpose and expected benefit of the treatment
- The likelihood of success
- The clinicians involved in their treatment
- The risks inherent in the procedure, however small the possibility of their occurrence, side effects and complications; the consequences of non-operative alternatives should also be explained
- Potential follow-up treatment.

Provided the patient is an adult with capacity, a Consent Form 1 should be completed. When filling out the form:

- Ensure legible writing
- Do not use abbreviations
- Detail the side and site and mark the patient accordingly if appropriate for the procedure.

3.3.2 COMPLEX CONSENT SITUATIONS

3.3.2.1 ADULT LACKING IN CAPACITY

It is necessary to ensure that a patient has capacity in order to give consent. Capacity can be established using the Mental Capacity Act 2005. Where a patient lacks capacity, the clinician should act in their best interests; this may require involving relatives that have lasting power of attorney or seeking second opinions from a consultant colleague.

Any advanced directive or living will completed whilst the patient still had capacity must be respected.

3.3.2.2 PAEDIATRIC PATIENTS

It is important to involve children in the consent process. As per the GMC guidelines:

- At 16, a young person can be presumed to have capacity to consent.
- A young person under 16 may have the capacity to consent depending on their maturity and ability to understand what is involved.

If a child is not deemed to have competence, consent must be obtained from at least one of the parents, or a person with legal responsibility for the child.

If parents refuse to give consent and this will lead to harm, for example, in the case of a Jehovah's witness not giving consent for their child to receive blood in the case of a post-tonsillectomy bleed, then the hospital legal team needs to be involved and the decision will be made in the patient's best interests.

In the case of an emergency, you may be asked to prepare the patient and consent for procedure prior to your senior arriving. The following details some specific examples of procedures that you may be required to consent for.

3.3.3 ARREST OF POST-TONSILLECTOMY BLEED

Indications: stop the active bleeding, prevent further bleeding and achieve haemodynamic stability

Risks: infection, bleeding (and return to theatre), pain, damage to teeth/lips/temporomandibular joint, taste disturbance, aspiration, need for blood transfusion

OPERATING THEATRE

3.3.4 MANIPULATION UNDER ANAESTHETIC OF FRACTURED NOSE

Indications: restore original nasal shape

Risks: infection, bleeding, pain, haematoma, residual deformity, nasal obstruction

3.3.5 MASTOIDECTOMY (ACUTE)

Indications: to clear infection and prevent complications of mastoiditis (e.g. meningitis, facial nerve palsy and intracerebral abscess)

Risks: infection, bleeding, scar, hearing loss (dead ear), tinnitus, dizziness, taste disturbance, facial nerve damage, CSF leak

3.3.6 TRACHEOSTOMY

Indications: these broadly fall into three categories: to relieve an obstructed upper airway, airway protection/management of respiratory secretions or need for prolonged intubation

Risks: airway compromise, infection, bleeding, scar, permanent tracheostomy, voice change, subcutaneous emphysema and tube dislodgement

3.3.7 DRAINAGE OF SEPTAL HAEMATOMA

Indications: reduce risk of infection, necrosis and nasal collapse

Risks: infection, bleeding (epistaxis), perforation of nasal septum and recurrence of haematoma

3.3.8 NASAL/EAR FOREIGN BODY REMOVAL

Indications: removal of foreign body

Risks: infection, bleeding, damage to surrounding structures (nasal cavity for nasal foreign bodies, tympanic membrane perforation or external ear canal abrasion for ear foreign bodies), aspiration (nasal foreign bodies)

OPERATING THEATRE

3.3.9 RIGID OESOPHAGOSCOPY (+/- REMOVAL FOREIGN BODY)

Indications: removal of foreign body (preventing further damage and perforation of oesophagus)

Risks: sore throat, damage to the teeth/lips/tongue/TMJ and mucosal or oesophageal tear, failure to remove

3.3.10 DRAINAGE OF PERIORBITAL ABSCESS

Indications: drain the abscess and treat the infection, preservation of sight

Risks: scar (if done via an external approach), infection, bleeding, pain, periorbital ecchymosis and emphysema, trauma to medial rectus muscle (endoscopic approach), epiphora (damage to nasolacrimal duct)

3.3.11 DEEP SPACE NECK ABSCESS

Indications: drain the abscess and treat the infection, prevent spread of infection (to mediastinum)

Risks: scar, infection, bleeding, damage to relevant neurovascular structures (depends on the location of the abscess: marginal mandibular nerve, lingual nerve, hypoglossal nerve, accessory nerve, recurrent laryngeal nerve, internal jugular vein or carotid artery), tracheostomy (in the event of airway compromise or failure to intubate), pneumothorax

3.3.12 SPA LIGATION

Indications: arrest of epistaxis

Risks: pain, infection, bleeding, palatal numbness (damage to nasopalatine nerve), risks of septoplasty (if required for access), failure to control bleeding requiring further procedures (further surgery/embolisation)

3.3.13 GROMMET INSERTION

Indications: allow drainage of pus from the middle ear

Risks: pain, infection, bleeding, residual perforation, early extrusion, need for further procedures, hearing loss (damage to the middle ear ossicles), inadvertent misplacement of grommet in the middle ear

OPERATING THEATRE

CHAPTER 4: WARD

4.1 POST-OP HEAD AND NECK PATIENTS

4.1.1 TYPES OF DRAIN

Surgical drains can be classified as open or closed – where a closed drain is a tube attached to a drainage pot. Another classification is active or passive, where passive is usually capillary action or gravity dependent and active has a negative pressure component. An example of a commonly used closed active system is a Redivac™ drain, in which a closed-tubed drain enters a bottle or bag under negative pressure, applying gentle continuous suction on the wound area to prevent liquid build up. When checking drains, it is important to document which side (if multiple drains), volume in the drain over 24 hours, and to check the seal/vacuum on the drain if it is a negative pressure drain.

4.1.2 FLAP CARE

Reconstructive flaps and grafts can be used in reconstruction, particularly during head and neck surgery. Grafts do not have an intrinsic blood supply and therefore monitoring of these is purely based on appearance of the graft.

Flaps by contrast come with a pedicled blood supply. A local or regional flap retains its original blood supply. A free flap is removed from its original site and is transplanted in a new site – microvascular reconstruction establishes a new blood supply through the pedicled vessels. Free flaps have many advantages including the potential donation of any tissue type and flexible size of graft. They do, however, need close post-operative monitoring, which will often be the job of the junior doctor on the ward. This can be done by monitoring graft capillary refill, colour, turgor and temperature, all of which should be similar to the surrounding skin. A hand-held Doppler can also check the flow through the feeding vessel and the operative surgeon will usually demonstrate or mark where to check this. Increasingly, implantable Doppler probes are being used. These are placed on the recipient vessel distal to the microsurgical anastomosis at the time of surgery to provide continuous monitoring in the immediate post-operative period. Operation notes will document frequency and type of checks needed and an escalation plan, but if there are any concerns, it is best to raise them early with a senior colleague.

4.1.3 PARENTERAL FEEDING

Dietetic input is required for all head and neck patients and should be instigated pre-operatively. An energy intake of 30 kcal/kg/day should be aimed for, with early tube feeding post-operatively and regular nutritional assessments. A gastrostomy should be considered if long-term feeding is likely to be required (over four weeks). Timing of feeding after laryngectomy will be determined by the operating surgeon, and the plan will be detailed in the operative notes – this may be done early, or delayed until after a post-operative swallow depending on the operative findings and the surgeon.

4.1.4 SWALLOWING ASSESSMENT

Speech and language therapists perform the majority of swallowing assessments conducted in hospital, which are primarily done by clinical assessment. They also perform fibre-optic endoscopic evaluation of swallowing (FEES), which they often do in conjunction with an ENT specialist. During FEES, different foods and drinks (often dyed) are ingested under endoscopic vision, and a sensory test (with puffs of air) is also performed.

During an ENT assessment of a head and neck patient, it is important to ask about aspiration symptoms (coughing and choking when eating or drinking) and recurrent chest infections. Any of these should warrant a speech and language review.

4.1.5 POST-OPERATIVE THYROID PATIENTS

Post-operative thyroidectomy patients can develop serious complications. One is a thyroid haematoma, where post-operatively the empty thyroid bed fills with blood and the accompanying swelling causes a reduction in venous return in the larynx – this causes congestion, oedema and narrowing of the airway. It is an airway emergency: the wound needs opening and the haematoma evacuating, which may need to be done acutely on the ward. Assess the patient's respiratory rate and oxygen saturations, and listen for stridor to assess how acutely this needs managing. Always involve a senior.

THE WARD

A more common complication after total (or completion) thyroidectomy is hypocalcaemia, caused by disruption or accidental removal of the parathyroid glands. Post-operative total or completion thyroidectomy patients should always have their calcium levels checked at both two and six hours post-operatively and should be monitored for symptoms such as perioral and fingertip paraesthesia. Those who are symptomatic or have an acute drop or severe hypocalcaemia (under 2.10 mmol/L) need a review, an ECG and IV calcium replacement. Check the British Association of Endocrine and Thyroid Surgeons (BAETS) guidelines and local trust guidelines for details on how to replace calcium.

4.1.6 TRACHEOSTOMY CARE

Patients may require a tracheostomy for airway obstruction, to manage upper respiratory tract secretions or to facilitate weaning from invasive ventilation. These can therefore be long term or temporary depending on the indication. Tracheostomy patients have an indwelling tracheostomy tube in their neck stoma, and these can be cuffed (which forms a definitive airway if cuff inflated) or uncuffed, and unfenestrated or fenestrated (facilitates upper airway air passage and voicing) (Figure 30). Most tracheostomy tubes have an inner and outer tube, where the inner tube can be removed for cleaning and then replaced. All tracheostomy patients will have a tracheostomy care pack next to the bed. Ask a local ENT nurse specialist or ENT senior colleague to show you a tracheostomy tube change – this will help with understanding and visualisation of the tracheostomy tube and stoma, and what to do in the case of tube dislodgment or blockage. The National Tracheostomy Safety Project (www.tracheostomy.org.uk) has some excellent resources, and all tracheostomy and laryngectomy patients should have a bed-end sign to demonstrate the type of tracheostomy they have. The basic anatomy is shown in Figure 24.

4.1.7 LARYNGECTOMY CARE

Laryngectomy patients have a neck stoma, but this is an end stoma (Figure 24). Any oxygenation or resuscitation must therefore occur through the neck stoma. They also do not typically have an indwelling tracheostomy tube long-term. A post-operative management plan will be detailed in the operation notes, as laryngectomy patients can have flaps that require monitoring, and may need post-operative calcium checks (if total thyroidectomy performed) and thyroxine prescribing.

THE WARD

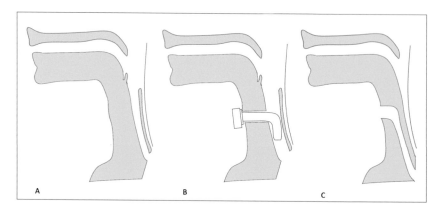

Figure 24: Diagram demonstrating: A) a patient with normal upper airways; B) a patient with a tracheostomy; and C) a laryngectomy patient. The important feature is the difference between tracheostomy and laryngectomy patient – the laryngectomy patient's stoma is not connected to either the nose or the mouth so they cannot be oxygenated via a face mask.

4.2 POST-OP RHINOLOGY PATIENTS

4.2.1 NASAL PACKS

Patients undergoing rhinology procedures such as FESS or septorhinoplasty may have nasal packs or splints inserted on completion of the procedure. Nasal packs may be absorbable, such as Nasopore®, or non-absorbable, such as Merocel® or Rapid Rhinos®. If the pack requires removal, the surgeon will leave instructions on when this should happen but if dissolvable, the patient should be informed that the pack will come out in pieces over the following few weeks. Patients are often encouraged to rinse their nose after such procedures, which will facilitate removal of dissolvable packs (check post-operative instructions for each patient).

4.2.2 NASAL SPLINTS

Nasal splints can be internal or external. Internal nasal splints are generally made of a soft and flexible material such as silicone. They are applied to either side of the septum with a suture through the septum. External nasal splints can be thermoplastic or plaster of Paris. These splints are usually removed after one week in the clinic (check surgeon's post-operative instructions).

4.2.3 PITUITARY PATIENTS

Most ENT departments that perform pituitary surgery have a protocol for managing post-operative patients that usually includes:

- Fluid balance monitoring and potentially fluid restriction
- U&Es, plasma osmolality, urine osmolality and glucose: monitoring for diabetes insipidus
- Steroids may be necessary if the patient develops diabetes insipidus
- On discharge, the patient should be advised to return if they notice clear fluid from their nose (CSF leak), severe headache or visual disturbance.

THE WARD

4.3 POST-OP OTOLOGY PATIENTS

4.3.1 HEAD BANDAGE AND DRESSINGS

Patients undergoing tympanomastoid surgery will often return from theatre with a head bandage and dressings placed over the operated ear. The length of time the bandage and external dressings need to be in place will vary and instructions for removal will be documented by the operating surgeon in the post-operative notes. Time frames vary from two hours to overnight and removal the following morning.

If an endaural or postaural approach has been used, sutures will be present. These may be absorbable or non-absorbable. The latter will require removal, usually by the patient's GP surgery, a week post-operatively.

4.3.2 PACKS

Patients will often have packing placed within the ear canal following surgery. This can be absorbable (e.g. Gelfoam® and Spongostan®) or non-absorbable (e.g. bismuth iodoform paraffin paste [BIPP] or a ribbon gauze coated in ointment containing antibiotic and steroid such as Terra-Cortri).

The absorbable packs do not usually need to be removed and patients are commonly given antibiotic drops (e.g. Ciloxan™) to apply topically for two-to-three weeks after the operation. Non-absorbable packs are typically kept in place for three weeks post-operatively and are removed by the surgeon in clinic when the patient is seen for review.

4.3.3 AFTERCARE

Following ear surgery, it is important that the patient keeps the ear dry to reduce the risk of infection. Patients should be instructed to take care when bathing and use cotton wool coated in petroleum jelly to ensure that water is kept from entering the ear canal. It is normal for there to be some slight bleeding from the ear for several days following the operation but this will slow down and stop. Patients are often advised to avoid forceful nose blowing and to sneeze with their mouths open for the first two weeks after surgery, as well as to avoid heavy lifting, strenuous exercise and excessive straining.

Patients who have undergone stapes surgery will often have specific instructions for strict bedrest initially, followed by slow mobilisation to reduce the risk of displacement of the prosthesis.

THE WARD

4.3.4 BASIC POST-OP CHECKS

The following should be checked in the post-operative period and before being discharged from the hospital. These should be documented in the notes and any abnormal findings escalated to your on-call senior:

- Check for facial nerve function
- Check for nystagmus
- Weber tuning fork test or the "scratch" test (if no tuning fork is available) – sound should localise to the operated ear
- Cochlear implant patients will often require a post-operative x-ray to check electrode placement. This will be specified in the post-operative instructions from the surgeon.

THE WARD

4.4 POST-OPERATIVE COMPLICATIONS

This section aims to give you more detail on post-operative complications that require urgent review. As a general principle, use the ABCDE approach and escalate to your senior team early. Surgeons audit their own surgical outcomes and complication rates, which may be included in your local morbidity and mortality meetings or even be part of a national audit. While the emergency is dealt with by the on-call team out-of-hours, it is important that the operating surgeon is made aware and involved in subsequent management of their patient the next day.

4.4.1 POST-TONSILLECTOMY OR POST-ADENOIDECTOMY BLEED

The oropharynx is highly vascular, supplied by branches of the external carotid artery (lingual, ascending pharyngeal, facial) and post-operative bleeding from tonsillectomy and to a lesser extent adenoidectomy can lead to significant and even life-threatening haemorrhage.

Primary haemorrhage is defined as a bleed occurring within the first post-operative day (<24 hours), while a secondary haemorrhage occurs after the first post-operative day (>24 hours).

Key points:

- ABCDE approach, obtain IV access and send of bloods (FBC, clotting, group and save +/- sample for crossmatch)
- Fluid resuscitation +/- blood transfusion as necessary
- Estimate and document the blood loss from the history of bleeding and clinical examination
- Ask patient to sit-up forwards and spit out blood and clots into a bowl to avoid risk of aspiration
- Consider the use of tranexamic acid IV (but bear in mind that at this point in time the evidence base for tranexamic acid use in post-tonsillectomy bleed is equivocal but is becoming more widespread; therefore, this should be discussed with your senior team)
- Do not attempt to remove clots in the tonsil fossa as these may be tamponading a bleeding vessel
- Adrenaline-soaked gauze on sponge holders applied to the actively bleeding tonsil fossa can be trialled but may not be well tolerated by the patient

THE WARD

- Escalate to your on-call senior and inform the anaesthetic team as actively bleeding cases may need transfer to theatres immediately from the emergency department
- Patients may have intermittent bleeding, or a small herald bleed prior to significant haemorrhage (common due to the arterial nature of post-tonsillectomy bleeds); therefore, do not be falsely reassured by the lack of active bleeding
- It is common practice to admit all post-tonsillectomy bleeds for a period of observation.

4.4.2 THYROID HAEMATOMA

A post-operative thyroid haematoma is a rare but significant complication due to the risk to the airway. Haematomas may present early, by compression and airway compromise due to an expanding haematoma, or later through the increased risk of post-op infection.

The patient is most at risk of a thyroid haematoma in the first 24 hours post-op (see section 4.1.5 on post-operative care of the thyroidectomy patient). There is no consensus on whether a drain is required post-thyroidectomy. Whether to insert a drain and what type of drain to use are dependent on the surgeon's technique and preference.

Red flags for a thyroid haematoma:

- Rapid increase in drain output (frank blood or heavy blood-stained fluid) or drain blockage
- Significant neck swelling post-op +/- patient reported pressure or discomfort
- Stridor and breathing difficulty (critical condition) – urgent haematoma drainage on ward required as a temporising measure.

Escalate to senior and perform decompression on ward in the presence of airway compromise.

Thyroid haematoma drainage:

Equipment: Headlight, gown/apron, gloves, sterile gauze, scalpel/scissors/staple-remover (depending on method of closure)

- Open the surgical wound at the surgical site (most important step)
- With a gloved finger, remove clots or haematoma if not sufficiently decompressed at time of opening the wound
- Transfer patient to theatre environment promptly for formal haematoma evacuation and arrest of bleeding under GA

THE WARD

4.4.3 OESOPHAGEAL PERFORATION

A serious complication of an oesophagoscopy procedure is oesophageal perforation. It leads to mediastinitis and sepsis, and must be treated promptly and aggressively. Patients who have oesophageal dilatation or instrumentation should be observed for a few hours post-procedure before discharge. The cardinal features of oesophageal perforation are chest pain (mainly felt on the back), fever and tachycardia. Surgical emphysema or signs of sepsis can also be seen in these patients. If perforation is suspected, the patient needs to be kept NBM and to be started on broad-spectrum antibiotics and IV fluids. If oesophageal perforation is suspected, inform the on-call senior. A CXR and possibly a CT scan of thorax will likely be required. A perforation may be managed conservatively or surgically, depending on the location and size.

4.4.4 EPISTAXIS AFTER NASAL SURGERY

Epistaxis after surgery is more complex to manage than simple epistaxis and should be escalated early. The risk after a septorhinoplasty or septoplasty is that the nasal and septal reconstruction that has occurred could be compromised after nasal packing, so other interventions such as good first aid should be trialled first (compression and ice). Epistaxis after FESS surgery can be profuse, and may need anterior or even posterior packing as there is a risk of damage to the sphenopalatine or anterior ethmoid arteries, although this would normally be diagnosed intraoperatively. If there is minimal bleeding, packing should be avoided if possible to avoid damage to the mucosal lining of the nose. However, as in all cases of epistaxis, if bleeding is profuse or life threatening then nasal packing is indicated. In septoplasty or septorhinoplasty cases, consider packing the nose bilaterally (even if the epistaxis is unilateral) if there is a chance that the high pressure from the nasal pack may move the septum (e.g. BIPP packing or a balloon nasal pack such as Rapid Rhino®). High-pressure unilateral packing in the early post-operative period could lead to septal deviation or dislocation. Call for senior assistance or advice early.

THE WARD

4.4.5 TRACHEOSTOMY TUBE DISPLACEMENT

Tracheostomy tubes can be displaced post-operatively. If this is after a week post-operatively, there will normally be a good, well-formed tract that the tracheostomy tube can easily be placed back in to. Prior to this, there is a chance of creating a false tract, so direct visualisation during replacement is crucial. Obtain senior support early if you don't have much experience with tracheostomies. If the situation is time critical, seek help from experienced nursing staff and the on-site anaesthetic team. Section 6.9 details the preparation and kit necessary for a tracheostomy tube change.

A good headlight, spare tracheostomy tube (the same size as the one dislodged and one the size smaller), suction, tracheostomy dilators and an assistant are required. Tracheal dilators can be placed in the tracheostomy stoma to open the site so that the tracheal rings (and tracheal window) can be seen to aid placement of the tube. Once the tube has been replaced, the placement into the trachea can be confirmed by using the nasendoscope through the tracheostomy tube. Oxygen saturations should be measured, and equal chest expansion/chest auscultation can confirm adequate ventilation.

THE WARD

CHAPTER 5: CLINIC

5.1 EMERGENCY CLINIC

Emergency ENT clinics are a vital aspect of all ENT departments and allow GPs, the emergency department and other non-ENT teams within the hospital to access specialist ENT care. The clinics are set up to allow assessment, diagnosis and management of common acute ENT conditions in an outpatient setting with appropriate equipment and senior support available. The clinics are normally run and managed by the junior doctors working within the ENT team, with senior support when required. Most clinics will run daily alongside main clinic and be appointment based, although some departments may operate an open-access/"walk-in" policy.

Conditions which are appropriate to be seen and managed in emergency clinic include the following:

- Otitis externa
- Otitis media
- Foreign bodies in the ear and nose
- Nasal fractures
- Pinna haematoma/abscess
- Recurrent epistaxis
- Acute facial palsy
- Sudden sensorineural hearing loss
- Acute TM perforation.

More acute conditions (e.g. airway emergencies) and those where admission may be required (e.g. tonsillitis, active epistaxis and peritonsillar abscess) should be seen and assessed in the emergency department. Other conditions such as an unexplained neck lump and persistent hoarseness (ongoing for over three weeks) should be referred via the suspected-head-and-neck-cancer pathway (two-week-wait pathway). More chronic conditions (ongoing for more than six weeks) such as hearing loss, recurrent ear/sinus/throat infections, nasal obstruction and dysphonia should be referred to the main clinic.

Each department will have guidelines for who should and shouldn't be seen in emergency clinic and these should be provided when commencing your ENT job.

5.2 MAIN ENT CLINIC

The majority of ENT patients are managed as outpatients and therefore clinics form a vital aspect of every ENT surgeon's day-to-day clinical activity. Patients are not only assessed but also managed as there are a number of procedures, both diagnostic and therapeutic, that are undertaken in the clinic setting. Clinics can be general or more subspecialised (e.g. balance clinic, two-week-wait clinics for suspected head-and-neck cancer, and voice clinics, amongst others). There are further details of subspecialist clinics in the following section.

THE CLINIC

5.3 SUBSPECIALIST ENT CLINICS

5.3.1 BALANCE CLINIC

This is a multidisciplinary clinic that usually consists of an ENT consultant, an audiologist and a balance therapist (physiotherapist). The balance system is made up of the vestibular system, visual input and proprioception. The term "dizziness" is non-specific and can describe anything from a feeling of light-headedness and unsteadiness to spinning. Vertigo is the sensation of rotation and this is how vestibular causes usually present along with other symptoms such as hearing loss, tinnitus and aural fullness. Central causes such as cerebellar pathology can also cause vertigo; however, associated symptoms are generally quite different – such as weakness, headache or dysarthria.

When assessing the patient, the MDT must firstly establish whether there is a vestibular element to the patient's symptoms and this is usually ascertained by taking a thorough history (Figure 23). Investigations may include pure-tone audiogram (PTA), MRI (if a central cause is suspected) and vestibular function tests (to characterise and quantify the patient's vestibular function).

5.3.2 HEAD AND NECK CLINIC

This is a multidisciplinary clinic that consists of an ENT head and neck consultant, a specialist head and neck cancer nurse, a dietician, and a speech and language therapist (SLT). In some centres, maxillofacial surgeons also contribute to the head and neck clinic. The role of this clinic is to see both new two-week waits and head-and-neck-cancer follow ups.

THE CLINIC

TWO-WEEK WAITS

- Patients who fit the following criteria can be referred to two-week-wait clinics (NHS England):
    - o An unexplained palpable lump in the neck that has changed over a period of 3–6 weeks
    - o Persistent unexplained hoarseness >3 weeks
    - o An unexplained persistent sore throat especially if associated with dysphagia, hoarseness or otalgia
    - o Persistent unilateral nasal obstruction with bloody discharge
    - o Unexplained unilateral serous otitis media/effusion in a patient >18.
- The patient will undergo a thorough clinical assessment and decisions will be made regarding further investigations such as imaging or upper aerodigestive tract endoscopy.

HEAD AND NECK CANCER FOLLOW-UP PATIENTS

- Patients should be followed up for a minimum of 5 years.
- Patients should be followed up at least 2 monthly for the first 2 years.
- Patients should be followed up at least 3–6 monthly for the subsequent 3 years.
- Clinical assessment should include adequate clinical examination, including fibre-optic rigid or flexible nasopharyngolaryngoscopy (BAHNO guidelines).

5.3.3 OTHER SPECIALIST CLINICS

5.3.3.1 COCHLEAR IMPLANT CLINIC

- This multidisciplinary clinic consists of ENT surgeons, Audiology, Teachers of the Deaf (paediatrics), and speech and language therapists (SLT).
- There are only a small number of centres that perform cochlear implantation in the UK.
- Patients who meet the criteria for cochlear implantation are referred to one of these centres.

THE CLINIC

- Assessment involves confirming that the patient still meets the criteria and ensuring that they have a realistic expectation of how life will be as a cochlear implant user and the commitment that they need to make to rehabilitation following implantation.

CRITERIA FOR COCHLEAR IMPLANTATION

- Paediatrics: simultaneous cochlear implantation is recommended in severe to profound hearing loss (defined as only hearing sounds that are louder than 80 dBHL at two or more frequencies in the range 500 Hz to 4 KHz bilaterally without acoustic hearing aids) patients who do not benefit from acoustic hearing aids (adequate benefit defined as speech, language and listening skills appropriate to age and development stage).
- Adults: unilateral cochlear implantation is recommended in severe to profound hearing loss patients who do not benefit from acoustic hearing aids (adequate benefit defined as a phenome score of 50 % or greater on the Authur Boothroyd word tests presented at 70 dBA).

5.3.3.2 VOICE CLINIC

- This MDT includes an ENT surgeon and SLT
- For patients with complex voice problems
- A thorough history will be taken including voice use and whether they suffer from acid reflux; Voice Handicap Index (VHI) and Reflex Symptom Index (RSI) scores are usually calculated
- Fibre-optic nasendoscopy is performed to identify pathology
- Stroboscopy may also be carried out, a technique in which a high-speed flashing light is combined with the flexible nasendoscopy. This provides a view of the vibrating vocal cords in slow motion. This technique provides more detailed information for the voice team and it can also be recorded to enable the patient to see the cause of their speech problems.

THE CLINIC

CHAPTER 6: PROCEDURES

6.1 NASAL CAUTERY

If conservative measures to stop epistaxis have failed, then nasal cautery can be a useful adjunct to treat epistaxis. Prepare the nose with local anaesthetic and a vasoconstrictor, ideally placing this on some cotton wool or gauze up the nose and leaving it for a few minutes – digital pressure can be applied over this to reduce bleeding.

- Using a headlight and a Thudichum nasal speculum, inspect the nasal septum – Little's area (Figure 3) is the most common source of bleeding.
- If a prominent vessel or bleeding point is identified, this may be cauterised. Using a silver nitrate stick, start surrounding the bleeding point and finishing centrally over the vessel. Apply saline-soaked gauze or a saline-soaked cotton-bud tip to the region and compress over this for a couple of minutes.
- Apply Naseptin cream (NOTE: this is made with peanut derivatives so check for allergies before use) and encourage patient to apply this gently for a week following cautery.
- Observe the patient for at least 20 minutes post-procedure to check for recurrent bleeding.
- Give epistaxis first-aid advice (described in section 2.9) and safety-net.

6.2 NASAL PACKING

Nasal packing is required if epistaxis cannot be controlled with first-aid measures or cautery. The patient needs to be informed of the next step and verbally consented for this, including explaining that the process of packing can be very uncomfortable.

Anterior nasal packing

- Using a headlight and a Thudichum nasal speculum, inspect the nose and suction out any clots.
- All acute epistaxis patients need IV access, a full set of bloods and fluid resuscitating as required. An assistant to suction blood and reassure the patient while you are packing a nose is invaluable.
- Prepare a nasal pack – normally either a Rapid Rhino® (inflatable balloon pack) or a Merocel® (dry sponge nasal tampon). A Rapid Rhino® needs removing from its blue sleeve and wetting with water; this activates the carboxymethyl cellulose layer to a lubricating gel. They also need inflating with air after placement so locate a 10 ml syringe. Merocels® need lubricant jelly applying.
- Both packs are inserted in the same manner – from anterior to posterior in a horizontal plane along the floor of the nose, i.e. not upwards (Figure 25). Lift the tip of the patient's nose with your non-dominant hand and aim the pack inferiorly and posteriorly and push the pack in with one smooth movement. The tip of the pack should just protrude from the nose, with the string or valve then taped to the patient's cheek. For a balloon pack, they should then be inflated with some air until the balloon cuff is inflated but not taut.
- If the bleeding doesn't stop, pack the contralateral side – this places increased pressure on the nasal septum.
- Reassess the patient's haemodynamic status and check the oropharynx for ongoing bleeding.
- Packing with ribbon gauze (either soaked in BIPP or paraffin) using a Tilley's nasal dressing forceps is an alternative means of nasal packing. Layer the ribbon in loops and pack all corners of the nasal cavity, both ends of the ribbon gauze should be kept out of the nose anteriorly. This is uncomfortable for the patient as it requires several passes with the dressing forceps but can be very effective.

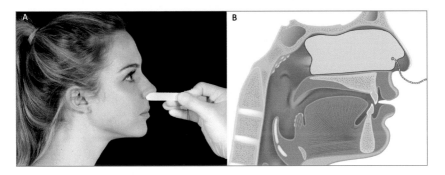

Figure 25: Insertion of anterior nasal pack (pack shown is a simple nasal tampon):
A – insertion angle for all packs; B – after inflation with saline (or air, if balloon pack),
pack fills nasal cavity and applies pressure for haemostasis.

Posterior nasal packing

- If the bleeding doesn't stop with bilateral packs in situ then call for senior assistance and consider a posterior pack on the original bleeding side. Rapid Rhino® do a longer pack with two balloons to inflate – this is worth considering as it offers some posterior packing.

- A posterior pack can be placed by use of a Foley catheter – the balloon tip end is passed into the postnasal space and inflated. You can confirm correct placement of the balloon by watching for the catheter in the oropharynx, inflating the balloon when the tip is seen and then retracting the catheter; it should sit snugly. Anterior packing is now required to secure the Foley catheter, and then the catheter is secured under some traction with an umbilical clip. The umbilical clip must not rest against the alar as it can cause alar necrosis. You can use a cut cuff of the Foley catheter or a pad to keep the clip away from direct pressure on the nostril – alert both the patient and the nursing staff to this.

- Reassess the patient's haemodynamic status and check the oropharynx for ongoing posterior bleeding.

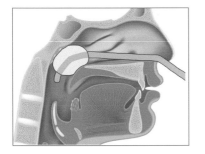

Figure 26: Posterior pack in the posterior choana. This would now require anterior packing and the catheter securing in order to complete the procedure.

PROCEDURES

6.3 QUINSY DRAINAGE

A quinsy is a peritonsillar abscess. In adults these can be drained through the mouth with the patient awake under local anaesthetic, either by needle aspiration or incision and drainage. Gain patient's verbal consent for the procedure (the main risks are bleeding and recurrence of the abscess collection). Spray the patient's oropharynx with local anaesthetic. If the patient has trismus then administering one dose of dexamethasone half an hour before drainage can help improve mouth opening. Locate a white (16G) needle and a 10 ml syringe. Prior to aspiration, label the depth of the needle, either with tape or by removing, cutting and replacing the needle cap, forming a "needle guard". Only 1 cm of needle should be proud, improving depth perception during aspiration.

- Using a headlight and a tongue depressor, inspect the patient's mouth, and identify the most prominent/bulging point of the abscess – this is where the needle or incision will be made.
- Spray local anaesthetic directly on this region.
- Needle aspiration can then be performed with a white needle. Up to three needle points can be aspirated (Figure 27). Alternatively, local anaesthetic can be injected and an incision made over the same site with a blade – only do this once someone has taught you how.
- You may need to use a smaller syringe (e.g. a 2 ml syringe) if you cannot pass a 10 ml syringe between the teeth due to trismus. Draining some pus will almost immediately improve trismus, allowing a larger syringe to be used.

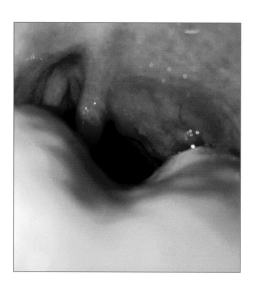

Figure 27: Quinsy, with recommended aspiration points marked by asterisk (*): three-point drainage can be attempted into the peritonsillar space.

PROCEDURES

6.4 PINNA HAEMATOMA

A pinna haematoma normally forms after shearing stress to the pinna or blunt trauma, but can also occur post-operatively. It needs drainage and this is best performed within 24 hours of injury. Sometimes these can be successfully aspirated, although there is a high risk of recollection, and an incision under local anaesthetic is the definitive treatment. In an out-of-hours emergency, aspiration can reduce the risk of avascular necrosis of the underlying cartilage, leaving the definitive treatment for the next day.

- Pinna skin should be cleaned with chlorhexidine or betadine and local anaesthetic infiltrated.

- Aspiration with a white needle (16G) on a 10 ml syringe or a curved incision can be placed adjacent to the helical rim. A dental roll or silastic splint should then be sutured down to prevent recollection – the suture to secure this is passed through and through the dental roll or splint and the pinna. A head bandage may then be placed over this to secure the dressings.

- A review at 48 hours is ideal to check for recollection. Sutures and rolls or splints can be removed then too.

- If there is a suggestion of contamination or abscess, commence oral antibiotics.

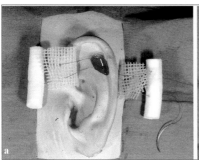 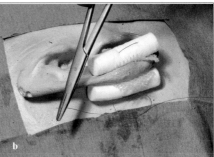

Figure 28: Pinna haematoma incision and dental roll application

PROCEDURES

6.5 SEPTAL HAEMATOMA DRAINAGE

This most commonly occurs as a result of trauma to the nose but can also happen post-operatively. Patients usually present after a fall or assault with nasal blockage and possibly nasal deviation.

> In any patient who presents to A&E with a nasal injury, ensure that you ask the referrer to assess for septal haematoma prior to discharging the patient. If present, the patient needs seeing acutely.

It can sometimes be difficult to differentiate between a septal haematoma and a nasal septal deviation just on inspection, so ensure you are using a headlight to free up your hands.

- Insert a Thudichum speculum into the nostril and, if you see a septal swelling (sometimes described as looking like a cherry), palpate it with a Jobson Horne probe to see if it is fluctuant. You can also use a gloved finger either side of the septum, which allows you to feel whether or not there is a collection present. (If there is a collection, it will feel fluctuant, whereas a deviated septum will feel firm to touch.)

- Once you have made the diagnosis of a septal haematoma, you need to arrange for incision and drainage under LA or GA. The longer the haematoma is left, the more likely it is to compromise the cartilage and lead to nasal deformity, so this should be arranged to be done ideally within 24 hours of onset.

- If you are unsure of the diagnosis, ask your senior to review the patient.

- Under LA or GA, infiltrate with local anaesthetic (e.g. Lignospan – 2 % lidnocaine with 1:80,000 adrenaline).

- Perform a vertical curved hemitransfixion incision of the septal mucosa and drain the blood/clot. If bilateral, this may all come out of one incision due to cartilage damage; if not, make bilateral incisions.

- Wash out the cavity with saline.

- If there is pus, send off an MC&S swab and consider inserting a small corrugated drain for 24 hours.

- Use a dissolvable suture such as Vicryl to quilt the septal mucosa (passing the needle back and forth through the mucosa and cartilage and tying it off on one side) – this will reduce risk of recurrence.

- If there are signs of infection, commence broad-spectrum antibiotics.

PROCEDURES

6.6 FLEXIBLE NASENDOSCOPY

This allows examination of the nasal cavity, pharynx, hypopharynx and larynx. Explain the nature of the procedure to the patient and confirm their consent verbally. See Figure 12 for a diagram of the scope.

- Apply topical local anaesthetic spray to the nose and oropharynx.
- Lubricate the end of the scope and introduce through the nose, along the floor, beneath the inferior turbinate.
- Advance the scope under direct vision to the postnasal space – assess the area including the presence of any masses, adenoidal tissue and the openings to the Eustachian tubes.
- Angle the scope inferiorly towards the oropharynx and ask the patient to breathe through the nose to keep the soft palate out of the way (Figure 29A). Guide the scope towards the oropharynx over the superior aspect of the soft palate.
- The posterior aspect of the palatine tonsils, tongue base, lingual tonsils and posterior pharyngeal wall can be viewed here (Figure 29B).
- Further advancement of the scope towards the larynx allows visualisation of the vallecula, epiglottis (lingual and laryngeal surface), aryepiglottic folds, piriform fossae and vocal cords (Figure 29C). Examination can be facilitated by asking the patient to protrude their tongue or performing a Valsalva manoeuvre. Vocal cord movement can be assessed by asking the patient to phonate (say "eeee" and count from 1 to 10).
- If the lens of the scope becomes obscured, ask the patient to swallow or brush the end of the lens gently against the mucosa to clear any secretions.
- Withdraw the scope in a controlled manner as this can also be very uncomfortable.
- Clean the scope in keeping with your hospital's decontamination protocol and document your findings.

PROCEDURES

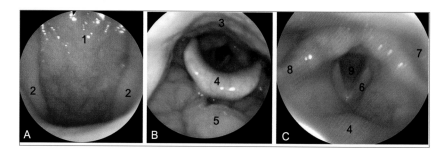

Figure 29: View of larynx on flexible nasendoscopy: A – view of postnasal space as patient inhales through nose; B – view of pharynx approaching larynx; C – view of larynx

1 – postnasal space; 2 – posterior eustachian tube cushion; 3 – posterior pharyngeal wall; 4 – epiglottis; 5 – base of tongue; 6 – left vocal cord (vocal fold); 7 – left piriform fossa; 8 – right aryepiglottic fold; 9 – laryngeal inlet/trachea

PROCEDURES

6.7 EAR MICROSUCTION

This is one of the most frequently performed procedures in the ENT outpatient clinic. It is generally performed for wax removal but can also be used for foreign body removal (section 6.8.2). When you first start your ENT job, try to visit the clinic and familiarise yourself with the microscope. Work out your inter-pupillary distance and how to control the zoom and focus. Your aim is to get a proper three-dimensional binocular vision.

- First examine the patient with an otoscope.
- Have the patient lying down with their head up at approximately a 45-degree angle.
- Ask them to turn their head away from the side you are microsuctioning to give a better view and insert an aural speculum into their ear.
- Inform them that they will hear a loud suctioning noise in their ear but that it shouldn't be uncomfortable.
- Suction out the wax, providing it is soft; this should come easily.
- If the wax is hard, the options are to use a wax hook to get behind the wax or, in cases where it is really impacted, the patient may need to use oil olive or sodium bicarbonate drops for a week prior to further attempts.

6.8 FOREIGN BODY REMOVAL

6.8.1 REMOVAL OF A NASAL FOREIGN BODY

A cooperative patient is essential to allow examination and successful removal. For younger children, parents and other staff members may be needed to position/support the child and provide reassurance. Topical vasoconstrictors are not normally indicated but can be applied to the nasal mucosa to improve access if there is a large amount of oedema present. Application of topical anaesthetics can improve patient's tolerance to instrumentation.

- **Direct instrumentation**
  - o This is the preferred method for easily visualised foreign bodies such beads and toys.
  - o Objects which are non-friable and non-spherical can be removed using Tilley or crocodile forceps.
  - o Instruments such as the wax hook are useful for spherical objects. The hook should be passed behind the object and the object then pulled forwards. Care should be taken not to damage the mucosa.
- **Balloon catheter**
  - o Small Foley catheters can be inserted past the object, the balloon inflated with 2–3 ml of air or water and the catheter pulled forwards to remove the foreign body.
- **Suction**
  - o A strong seal is needed to remove more solid foreign bodies. Flexible suction catheters are relatively atraumatic and can be used in young children, especially when dealing with organic foreign bodies that cannot be grasped.
- **Positive pressure**
  - o In children who are old enough, a forced exhalation method can be used by asking the child to blow hard through the nose whilst occluding the unaffected nostril.
  - o In younger children, the "Mother's Kiss" method can be used. The parent is asked to form a seal with their mouth over their child's mouth, occlude the unaffected nostril and give a short sharp blow.

PROCEDURES

- **Magnets**
  - o These can be used for small metallic objects such as button batteries and ball bearings.

6.8.2 REMOVAL OF AN EAR FOREIGN BODY

Various techniques can be used to remove ear foreign bodies from the external ear canal (either using a headlight and ear speculum or using the microscope) as follows:

- **Suction**
  - o Suction can be used to remove foreign bodies from the ear canal and also to remove any discharge present to allow better visualisation.
- **Mechanical instrumentation**
  - o Foreign bodies such as cotton wool and hearing-aid inserts can be removed using crocodile forceps.
  - o Spherical objects such as beads may require use of a wax hook or Jobson Horne probe. These instruments need to be passed behind the object and then withdrawn to allow removal.
- **Irrigation**
  - o Can be used to wash the foreign body out and should be used in combination with suction.
  - o This should be avoided if there is a perforation present as irrigation may dislodge the foreign body into the middle ear, predisposing the patient to infection and cause pain.

6.8.3 REMOVAL OF AN OROPHARYNGEAL FOREIGN BODY

More common in adults, this is generally caused by a fish bone or a small chicken bone. Take the history from the patient, asking exactly where they feel the foreign body (FB) and what they think it is. An x-ray can be obtained by A&E prior to referral; however, a lot of fish bones are not radio-opaque. The majority of fish bones are found in the tonsils, base of tongue or vallecula.

You will need local anaesthetic spray, a headlight, a flexible nasendoscope and possibly a rigid endoscope. Examine the patient both intra orally and with flexible nasendoscopy to ascertain where the FB is.

PROCEDURES

If the FB is in the tonsils and visible on oral examination, it can usually just be removed with a pair of Tilley forceps. If the FB is lodged in the base of tongue/vallecula it may require two people to remove it:

- One person will need to grip the patient's tongue firmly in a swab and pull it outwards. Their other hand should be free to grasp the FB with paediatric Magill forceps, fish-bone forceps or Tilley forceps.
- The other person will pass the flexible nasendoscope to visualise the FB, ideally with a stack system so everyone can see.
- Using a 30-degree rigid endoscope through the mouth instead of an FNE can be very useful too.
- If neither of these techniques is successful then the patient will require a GA for removal.

6.9 CHANGING A TRACHEOSTOMY TUBE

It is important to understand how a tracheostomy is performed in order to be able to change a tube safely (see section 4.4.5). You should not be asked to perform a tracheostomy change alone if you have not done it before and should seek assistance from senior members of the team if you are unsure.

Indications

- First tube change (usually seven days following insertion of a surgical tracheostomy)
- Established tracheostomies – change at 30 days (as per most manufacturer recommendations)
- Change in type of tube – e.g. change of a cuffed non-fenestrated tube for an uncuffed fenestrated tube
- Improve fit
- Replace a misplaced or faulty tube

In the case of a first tube change, caution needs to be exercised. This is also the case where previous difficult tube changes have been documented or the patient has excessive granulation tissue surrounding their stoma. If it is anticipated that the tube change will be challenging then it should be performed by an experienced clinician. Even in patients where the tube change is thought to be routine, it is recommended that two competent practitioners perform the procedure together.

Equipment required:

- Headlight
- Dressing pack
- Tracheostomy tubes of suitable size and one size smaller, with tapes/ties
- Tracheal dilators
- 10 ml syringe (if removing or inserting a cuffed tracheostomy tube)
- Suction and suction catheters
- Water-based lubricating gel
- Stoma dressing
- Stitch cutter if removing sutures (in case of first tube change)
- Gloves, apron, mask and visor

Tracheostomy tube changes can be performed "blind" or using a guide. The former is used more commonly and in the presence of an established tract. A guide such as a gum elastic bougie may be used if a difficult tube change is anticipated.

PROCEDURES

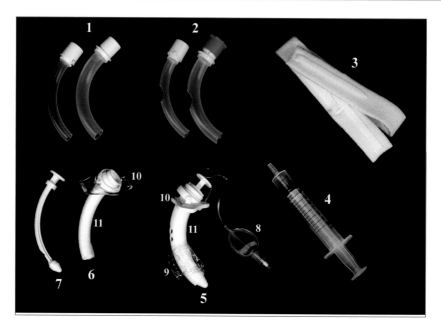

Figure 30: Tracheostomy tubes: 1 – inner tube; 2 – fenestrated inner tube (facilitates voicing); 3 – neck straps; 4 – 10 ml syringe to inflate cuff; 5 – fenestrated cuffed tracheostomy tube with introducer inserted; 6 – uncuffed non-fenestrated tracheostomy tube without introducer; 7 – introducer (obturator) alone; 8 – tracheostomy cuff inflation port; 9 – cuff; 10 – flange; 11 – fenestrations (holes)

PROCEDURE

BENEFITS
- To change tracheostomy tube
- Maintain patent and healthy stoma

RISKS
- Infection
- Bleeding
- Granulations
- Misplacement and creation of a false passage (surgical emphysema, pneumothorax/pneumomediastinum)
- Airway obstruction

PROCEDURE

- Explain the procedure to the patient and obtain verbal consent.
- Check all equipment is ready, check balloon on tube if inserting a cuffed tube.
- Lubricate the new tube and insert the introducer (obturator). (The introducer is not required if using a guided technique.)
- Set up the suction.
- Position the patient with the neck extended. Pillows or a roll under the shoulders may help.
- Check for sutures and remove them with a stitch cutter.
- Perform suction.
- Deflate cuff.
- Hold tube firmly in place and undo tape/ties.
- If using a guided technique, insert the bougie/guide.
- Remove the existing tube as the patient exhales.
- Insert the new tube, holding the introducer in place, and insert into the stoma. For a guided technique, insert the tube over the guide and through the stoma.
- Remove the introducer/guide.
- Check correct position by asking patient to breathe in and out. Air should be felt at the end of the tube.
- Inflate cuff (if required).
- Secure tube with tapes/ties and insert stoma dressing.

Reference: National Tracheostomy Safety Project (NTSP):
www.tracheostomy.org.uk

PROCEDURES

6.10 LARYNGECTOMY PATIENT SPEAKING VALVES

Laryngectomy speaking valves – or TEP (transoesophageal puncture) voice prostheses – are used by patients to produce speech. The specialised one-way valve sits in a hole in the posterior tracheal wall between the trachea and the oesophagus (Figure 31). The puncture is often performed as a primary procedure at the time of laryngectomy or as a secondary procedure several weeks after the initial operation. Temporary occlusion of the stoma allows exhaled air from the trachea to be diverted through the valve into the oesophagus. Vibrations in the oesophageal wall are used to create speech.

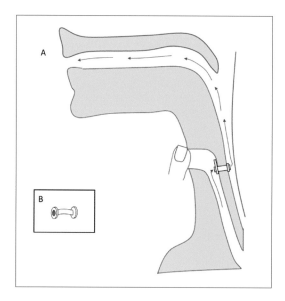

Figure 31: Laryngectomy patient demonstrating direction of airflow (A) and speech valve (B)

PROCEDURES

Speaking valves are normally inserted and changed by head and neck clinical nurse specialists and speech and language therapists. You may be asked to see a patient with a valve problem if they attend as an emergency, usually because the valve has come out or become dislodged. In such situations it is sensible to ask for senior support.

If the valve is out and a new one cannot be inserted, a Foley catheter or NGT of a suitable size should be used to keep the puncture patent and the patient can re-attend during working hours to have the valve re-inserted by trained staff. If the location of the TEP valve is not known and there is a possibility that it could have fallen into the airway, an FNE and chest x-ray should be performed and the above steps taken to keep the puncture patent. Senior help should be sought.

6.11 NERVE BLOCKS OF THE NOSE AND PINNA

Peripheral nerve blocks are a useful way of providing localised anaesthesia to areas of the head and neck when performing minor procedures in clinic and in the emergency department. From an ENT perspective, the most useful nerve blocks are those for the nose and pinna. In general, nerve blocks of the face (for example, supraorbital, supratrochlear, infraorbital and mental nerve blockade) will be utilised more by the Oral and Maxillofacial team when repairing lacerations.

Anaesthesia of the nose

Anaesthesia of the nose can be obtained using topical sprays, local injections and regional blocks, depending on the indication. A clear idea of the anatomy of nasal innervation is important. The main supply of the external nose is from the ophthalmic (V1) and maxillary (V2) divisions of the trigeminal nerve. The supratrochlear (V1), infratrochlear (V1) and external nasal branch of the anterior ethmoid nerve (V1) supply the superior part of the nose as well as the nasal tip. The lateral and inferior parts of the nose (including the lower eyelids) are supplied by the infraorbital nerve (V2) (Figure 32).

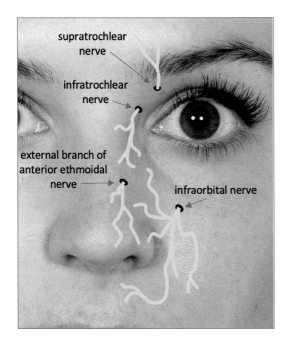

supratrochlear nerve

infratrochlear nerve

external branch of anterior ethmoidal nerve

infraorbital nerve

Figure 32: Sensory nerve supply to the external nose

PROCEDURES

The internal nose is also supplied by branches originating from the trigeminal nerve. The majority of the septum is supplied by the anterior and posterior ethmoid nerves (V1) as well as the nasopalatine nerve (V2) from the sphenopalatine ganglion.

Indications for use of local nasal anaesthesia:

- External nose
    - o Reduction of a nasal fracture
    - o Wound repair
    - o Drainage of an abscess
- Internal nose
    - o Examination of the nose, including nasendoscopy
    - o Drainage of septal haematoma
    - o Removal of a foreign body
    - o Nasal packing
    - o Nasal cautery

Equipment (depends on procedure) may include:

- Headlight
- Local anaesthetic (see below)
- Cotton wool or neuropatties
- Tilley forceps
- Dental syringe and needle (or alternatively, a 5 ml syringe with a 25G to 30G needle)
- Skin preparation (e.g. alcohol wipe for nasal fracture or betadine/chlorhexidine for wounds)
- Suture kit and appropriate sutures (e.g. 5-0 Prolene)

Anaesthetic agents (always check patient's allergy status):

- Topical anaesthetics
    - o Lidocaine hydrochloride (5 %) with phenylephrine hydrochloride (0.5 %) (co-phenylcaine) (for aged 12 years and over)
    - o Lidocaine 5 %
- Local infiltration
    - o Lignospan Special (lidocaine hydrochloride 2 % and adrenaline 1:80,000)
    - o Lidocaine 1 % (with or without adrenaline)

- Nerve block

    o   Lidocaine 1 %

    o   Bupivacaine 0.5 %

Technique:

For internal nasal anaesthesia, anaesthetic solutions can be sprayed or applied on cotton wool or neuropatties. Application of a nasal decongestant such as xylometazoline hydrochloride (Otrivine®) can be helpful prior to applying the local anaesthetic.

For the external nose, in the case of nasal fractures, local anaesthetic should be injected along the dorsum and laterally along the nasal bones. For other procedures such as wound closure, injection of anaesthetic will need to be tailored according to the location of the injury.

Infraorbital nerve blocks can be performed via various approaches:

- Percutaneously – inject 1 cm below the orbital rim in the mid-pupillary line down to the bone
- Intranasally – through the nasal vestibule into the facial soft tissue laterally, aiming 1 cm below the orbital rim in the midline
- Intraorally – via the buccal mucosa of the inner upper lip whilst palpating for the infraorbital foramen.

Remember always to aspirate prior to injecting the anaesthetic (to ensure you are not in a vessel) and infiltrate whilst withdrawing the needle.

Complications:

    o   Pain and discomfort at site of application

    o   Bleeding

    o   Infection

    o   Neuropraxia

    o   Toxicity (amount of anaesthesia used should not exceed maximal doses)

    o   Adverse effects of adrenaline (tachycardia, hypertension etc.)

Anaesthesia of the ear

The external ear is supplied by the auriculotemporal nerve, lesser occipital nerve, greater auricular nerve and the auricular branch of the vagus nerve. The external ear canal is supplied by the auriculotemporal nerve, auricular branch of the vagus nerve and the facial nerve.

PROCEDURES

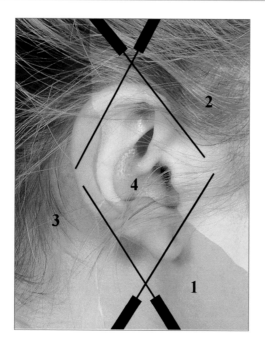

Figure 33: Sensory nerve supply to the pinna: 1 – greater auricular nerve; 2 – auriculotemporal nerve; 3 – lesser occipital nerve; 4 – auricular branch of vagus nerve; the needles indicate placement for nerve block of entire pinna.

Indications for use of local ear anaesthesia:

- Incision and drainage of pinna abscess
- Incision and drainage of pinna haematoma
- Closure of laceration of the pinna

Equipment (depending on procedure) may include:

- Headlight
- Local anaesthetic (see below)
- Dental syringe and needle (or alternatively, a 5 or 10 ml syringe with a 25G to 30G needle)
- Skin preparation (betadine/chlorhexidine for wounds)
- Scalpel
- Suture kit and appropriate sutures (e.g. 4-0 Vicryl, 5-0 Prolene)
- Corrugated drain and splints (for abscess/haematoma)
- Head bandage/other dressings

Anaesthetic agents (always check the patient's allergy status):

- Lignospan Special (lidocaine hydrochloride 2 % and adrenaline 1:80,000)
- Lidocaine 1 % (with or without adrenaline)
- Bupivacaine 0.5 %

PROCEDURES

Technique:

A ring block can be performed to provide anaesthesia to the whole ear (excluding the concha and external ear canal) (Figure 33). With this technique the injection needs to occur just under the skin around the pinna and not into the ear itself.

For small lacerations, a localised injection surrounding the area of injury may be more appropriate.

Remember always to aspirate prior to injecting the anaesthetic (to ensure you are not in a vessel) and infiltrate whilst withdrawing the needle.

Complications:

As per nasal anaesthesia

6.12 MANIPULATION UNDER ANAESTHETIC (MUA) FRACTURED NOSE

When patients are referred acutely with a fractured nose, remember to confirm the referrer has excluded a septal haematoma, as this requires a same-day review. If post-traumatic nasal deformity is suspected, the patient needs to be seen by the ENT team to assess the nasal skeleton after five-to-seven days. This allows the initial swelling to settle so bony deformities can be better assessed. The manipulation can occur up to 14 days post fracture, and can be done under local or general anaesthetic. The technique is shown above.

Once the patient has been consented, a nasal block can be performed with local anaesthetic (see section 6.11). Lie the patient supine on a couch so that you can access the couch from the head-end. Using thumbs bilaterally, digital pressure is applied over the nasal bones to push the nasal bones back into a more normal position. Often an audible/palpable crack occurs. No dressings are required unless the nasal bones are felt to be unstable, in which case a splint can be applied.

PROCEDURES

6.13 CRICOTHYROIDOTOMY

Cricothyroidotomy should be performed if there is an emergency airway situation where the team cannot oxygenate (intubate) or ventilate the patient. Figure 34 demonstrates the anatomical location of the cricothyroid membrane, the location at which this is performed. Figure 35 is taken from the Difficult Airway Society (DAS) guidelines and demonstrates the steps taken to perform this procedure.

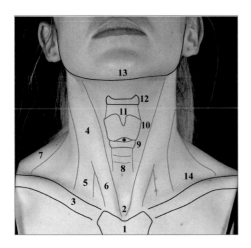

Figure 34: Neck image demonstrating location of cricothyroidotomy incision site (black asterisk *): 1 – sternum; 2 – suprasternal notch; 3 – clavicle; 4 – sternocleidomastoid (SCM); 5 – cleidomastoid part SCM; 6 – sternomastoid part SCM; 7 – trapezius; 8 – trachea; 9 – cricoid; 10 – thyroid cartilage; 11 – thyrohyoid membrane; 12 – hyoid; 13 – mentum; 14 supraclavicular fossa; * – cricothyroid membrane

PROCEDURES

Failed intubation, failed oxygenation in the paralysed, anaesthetised patient

2015

CALL FOR HELP

Continue 100% O₂
Declare CICO

Plan D: Emergency front of neck access

Continue to give oxygen via upper airway
Ensure neuromuscular blockade
Position patient to extend neck

Scalpel cricothyroidotomy

Equipment: 1. Scalpel (number 10 blade)
2. Bougie
3. Tube (cuffed 6.0mm ID)

Laryngeal handshake to identify cricothyroid membrane

Palpable cricothyroid membrane
Transverse stab incision through cricothyroid membrane
Turn blade through 90° (sharp edge caudally)
Slide coude tip of bougie along blade into trachea
Railroad lubricated 6.0mm cuffed tracheal tube into trachea
Ventilate, inflate cuff and confirm position with capnography
Secure tube

Impalpable cricothyroid membrane
Make an 8-10cm vertical skin incision, caudad to cephalad
Use blunt dissection with fingers of both hands to separate tissues
Identify and stabilise the larynx
Proceed with technique for palpable cricothyroid membrane as above

Post-operative care and follow up
• Postpone surgery unless immediately life threatening
• Urgent surgical review of cricothyroidotomy site
• Document and follow up as in main flow chart

This flowchart forms part of the DAS Guidelines for unanticipated difficult intubation in adults 2015 and should be used in conjunction with the text.

Figure 35: Performing a scalpel cricothyroidotomy from the Difficult Airway Society
https://das.uk.com

PROCEDURES

AUTHOR BIOGRAPHIES

Hannah Nieto BSc, MBBS, MRCS, PhD is an academic clinical lecturer in ENT in the West Midlands with an interest in bioinformatics, thyroid research and teaching.

Katherine McNamara MBChB, PGCert, FRCS(ORL-HNS) is an ENT ST8 in the West Midlands. She has a particular interest in education. She has completed an Education PGCert, runs a biannual ENT emergency course and is faculty on a number of other trainee courses.

Samantha Goh BA, MA(Cantab), MBBS, PGDip (MedEd), MRCS(ENT) is a senior higher specialty trainee who is passionate about global surgery and education. She organises the West Midlands Introduction to ENT Emergencies course and is currently a digital surgical teaching fellow in the West Midlands, developing a postgraduate virtual learning environment for core and higher surgical training.

Nina Mistry BSc(Hons), MBChB(Hons), MD(Res), FRCS(ORL-HNS) is a post-CCT Otology fellow currently working at Gloucester Royal Hospital and has been appointed as an ENT consultant at Worcestershire Acute Hospitals NHS Trust. She has a keen interest in teaching and training and has taught on several courses for junior doctors. Nina is also the digital education lead for the Student and Foundation Doctors in Otolaryngology (SFO-UK) committee, which aims to raise awareness of ENT as a career and promotes education in the field.

Shahram Anari MD, MSc, FRCS(ORL-HNS) is an ENT consultant working at University Hospitals Birmingham NHS Foundation Trust. He works as a rhinologist and facial plastic surgeon with a subspecialist interest in rhinoplasty and nasal reconstruction. He is actively involved in teaching and regularly teaches on different courses.

BIBLIOGRAPHY

Advanced Life Support from the Resuscitation Council UK: www.resus.org.uk

British Association of Endocrine and Thyroid Surgeons (BAETS): www.baets.org.uk

Difficult Airway Society guidelines: das.uk.com

European Position Paper on Rhinosinusitis and Nasal Polyps: www.rhinologyjournal.com

National Confidential Enquiry into Patient Outcome and Death (NCEPOD): www.ncepod.org.uk

National Tracheostomy Safety Project (NTSP): www.tracheostomy.org.uk

NICE guidelines: www.nice.org.uk

Scottish Intercollegiate Guidelines Network: www.sign.ac.uk

INDEX

acetic acid   33, 35, 88
acute mastoidectomy   112
acute mastoiditis   39, 82–4
acute otitis media (AOM)   4, 34, 35, 68, 78–81, 83, 92
acute rhinosinusitis   38, 66–7
acute sialadenitis   60–1
acute vertigo   91–3
adrenaline nebuliser   43, 46, 52
airway emergency   43, 45–7, 52, 54, 58, 105, 116, 123, 127, 155–6
airway examination   23–4
allergic rhinitis   36, 37, 38
aryepiglottic fold   139, 140
audiometry   30, 75, 92, 94
Avamys®   37
azelastine hydrochloride   36

balance clinic   128–9
balloon catheter   142
barium swallow   57, 102, 104
Beconase®   36
betametasone   33
Betnesol®   36
BIPP   35, 41, 63, 120, 124, 134
blunt neck trauma   103–4
Brodsky tonsillar grading   48
budesonide   43, 46, 52
button batteries   70, 72, 143

capacity   110–11
Cetraxal®   34
chronic rhinosinusitis   36–7, 67
chronic sinusitis   38
Cilodex®   34
Ciloxan®   34, 120
ciprofloxacin   34, 40, 90, 96
clinic   4, 15–24, 127–31, 141
clioquinol   34
clotrimazole   34, 88
cochlear implant   108, 121, 130–1
conductive hearing loss   30–1, 76, 95, 99
consent   110–13
cricothyroidotomy   46, 47, 155–6

deep space neck abscess   113
dexamethasone   34, 35, 42, 46, 49, 51, 52, 136
Difficult Airway Society   xi, 46–7, 155–6
drains   46, 59, 65, 105, 112–13, 115, 123, 136, 137, 138, 150, 152
Dymista®   37
dysphagia   13, 25, 48, 52, 54, 56, 57, 89, 90, 101, 103, 130
dysphonia   13, 54, 101, 103, 127

ear foreign body (or aural foreign body)   4, 72–3, 112, 143
EarCalm®   33, 88
emergency clinic   4, 77, 88, 97, 127
endoscopic sinus surgery   67, 107
epiglottis   26, 52, 139, 140
epiglottitis   4, 23, 45, 52–3
epistaxis   4, 6, 13, 38, 41, 62–3, 70, 98, 112, 113, 124, 127, 133, 134
ethmoid sinus   64
external auditory canal   8, 85–6, 88, 89, 99

facial nerve   7–8, 12, 16, 29, 42, 75, 90, 99–100, 108, 121, 151
facial nerve palsy   4, 7, 68–9, 82, 83, 100, 112
facial trauma   4, 97–8
flaps   3, 115–16, 117
flexible nasendoscopy   6, 19, 22–3, 46, 51, 52, 56, 101, 103, 130, 131, 140, 143
Flixonase®   37
Floseal®   41
flumetasone   34
fluticasone   37
foreign body, neck   23, 26–7, 56–7, 105, 107, 113, 143–4
fractured nose   4, 97, 98, 106, 112, 154
framycetin sulphate   35
free field hearing tests   16–18
frontal sinus   28, 64

functional endoscopic sinus
    surgery   67, 107

gastro-oesophageal reflux   13, 78
gentamicin   34
Genticin®   34
Gentisone-HC®   34
grommet   15, 32, 74, 83, 113

Haemophilus influenza   48, 52, 78
head and neck   3, 9, 14, 115, 116,
    129–30
head bandage   120, 137, 152
head injury   74, 75, 94, 97–100
hearing loss   4, 13, 17–18, 30–1, 42, 72,
    75, 79, 82, 86, 89, 91, 94–5, 99, 112,
    127, 129, 131
heliox   43
House–Brackmann grading   68–9, 99,
    100
hyperthyroidism   20–1, 35
hypothyroidism   21

incus   8, 29, 74
inner tube   117, 146
ipratropium bromide   38

Kiesselbach's plexus   6

laryngectomy   116–18, 148
lasers   108–9
lateral soft tissue neck   25–6
Little's area   6, 133
Locorten-Vioform®   34
Ludwig's angina   4, 23, 45, 59

magnets   143
malleus   8, 9, 29, 74
manipulation under anaesthetic of
    fractured nose   97, 112, 154
maxillary sinus   28
Merocel®   40, 63, 119, 134
microscope   64, 73, 96, 107–8, 141, 143
microsuction   75, 76, 86, 87, 88, 90,
    107, 141
middle ear   7–9, 15–16, 29–32, 78, 79,
    82, 107–9, 113, 143
mometasone furoate   37
myringoplasty   76, 83

nasal cautery   62, 63, 133, 134, 150
nasal foreign body   4, 70–1, 112, 142
nasal packing   40–1, 98, 119, 124,
    134–5, 150
nasal splints   119, 154
Nasonex®   37
Nasopore®   41, 119
NCEPOD   105–6
nebuliser   43, 52
neck examination   18–20, 23, 54
neck lump   4, 13, 19, 54–5, 127
neck lymph nodes   9–10, 20, 48
necrotising otitis externa   40, 85,
    88–9
neomycin   33, 35
nerve blocks   149–53
nerve monitor   108

odynophagia   13, 48, 50, 52, 101
oesophageal foreign body   56–7, 113
oesophageal perforation   56–7, 113,
    124
olive oil   34, 72
operating theatre   105–13
oral cavity   12, 18, 23, 48, 54
otalgia   13, 48, 50, 72, 75, 79, 82, 86,
    89, 130
otitis externa   4, 33–5, 40, 85–9, 96,
    127
Otocomb Otic®   35
Otomize®   35
otorrhoea   13, 75, 80, 89
Otosporin®   35
Otrivine®   38, 66, 151

paediatric patients   27, 33, 36, 39, 52,
    70, 80–1, 111, 130, 131
paranasal sinuses   7, 27–8, 66
parathyroid   10, 11, 117
parenteral feeling   116
parotid duct   8
parotid gland   7, 11, 12, 20, 55, 60
penetrating neck trauma   101–2
perichondritis   96
periorbital cellulitis   4, 64–5
pinna   15, 72, 82, 85, 86, 96–8, 137,
    149, 152–3
pinna haematoma   97–8, 127, 137, 152
piriform fossa/-ae   27, 56, 139, 140

pituitary   3, 11, 119
post-tonsillectomy bleed   111, 122–3
prednisolone   42, 68, 95
pseudomonas aeruginosa   76, 78, 85, 89, 96

quinsy   4, 49–51, 136
quinsy drainage   136

Rapid Rhino®   41, 63, 119, 124, 134–5
regional blocks   149
Rinatec®   38
Rinne   16–17

saline nasal douche   38–9, 66
semicircular canal   8, 29
sensorineural hearing loss   17, 30–1, 42, 94–5, 99, 127
septal haematoma   97, 98, 105, 112, 138, 150, 154
sodium bicarbonate   34, 141
sodium cromoglicate   36
Sofradex®   35
speaking valve   148
sphenopalatine artery ligation   113
stapes   8, 74, 120
stertor   24, 45
streptococcus pneumoniae   78
stridor   4, 24, 43, 45, 51, 52, 101, 116, 123
submandibular glands   11–12, 20, 58, 60
sudden-onset hearing loss   94–5
surface anatomy   5, 9
swallowing   19, 20, 54, 56, 58, 90, 116, 139

temporal bone   7, 28–9, 75, 83, 89, 95
temporal bone fracture   4, 76, 97, 99
thyroid examination   18, 19, 20–1
thyroid gland   10–11, 20
thyroid haematoma   4, 116, 123
thyroidectomy   45, 116–17, 123
thyroxine   10, 117
Tilley forceps   71, 134, 142, 144, 150
tinnitus   13, 75, 86, 112, 129
tonsillitis   4, 39, 48–9, 50, 51, 127
trachea   11, 24, 45, 103, 125, 140, 148, 155
tracheostomy   46–7, 59, 105, 107, 112, 113, 117–18
tracheostomy tube change   117, 125, 145–7
Tri-Adcortyl Otic®   35, 88
Trimovate®   35
tuning fork   16–17, 94, 121
two-week wait   127–30
tympanic membrane perforation   32, 72, 74–7, 79, 82, 83, 88, 99, 112
tympanometry/tympanograms   31–2, 75, 94
tympanoplasty   77, 107, 108

vertigo   4, 13, 16, 89, 99, 129
acute vertigo   91–3
vocal cord   45, 52, 131, 139–40
voice clinic   128, 131

Weber   16–17, 121

xylometazoline   38, 151